LIFE PROLONGING AND HEALTH PROMOTING LIFESTYLE

Dr. Thomas A. MaccAfi (MBBS)

© 2021 by Dr. Thomas A. MaccAfi (MBBS)

ISBN: 9798730179950

Published in Nigeria by:

Nkanemi Services

Nkanemiservices@gmail.com

CONTENTSPage

ACKNOWLEDGMENT

I am eternally thankful to my late wife, Martha and my five children Atari, Eugene, Ollu David, Joy and Rita, for bearing patiently through the years I have worked on this book. I have unavoidably denied them so much quality time and comfort enjoyed by their peers.

I am also very grateful to Professor A.C. Ikeme, (MD, FRCP, WHO Consultant) of the Foundation Clinic, Jos, for taking time off his very busy schedule to read through and correct the original manuscript.

I wish to use this page to express my profound gratitude to the following friends who have stood by me through thick and thin, both morally and financially, throughout the preparation of the book. They are: Mr. and Mrs. Yinka Owoborode, Mr. and Mrs. Charles Wilcox, Alhaji Ahmed Mu'azu and family, Late Senator E.N. Aboki, Mr. and Mrs. J.A. Akku, Mr. and Mrs. Abdullahi of Bevelyns Restaurant, Dr. Tunji Yusufof New Era Hospital Jos, and Mr. and Mrs. MikeLonghoom of Moriya Printing Press. Their contributions were simply priceless.

I willalso like to sincerely thank Mr. and Mrs. Adeolu Bilewu and all the staff of VT. Computers Jos for their patience and exemplary commitment to excellence.

I would want to use this opportunity to remember with deep appreciation the part played by my late friend and manager, Mr. Silvanus Isa, who retrieved the old copy of the manuscript, dusted it and worked day and night to retype it but could not live to see the published work. May his gentle soul rest in peace.

I also wish to acknowledge the invaluable contribution of my editor, Mr. Gilbert Edoreh, who worked tirelessly and meticulously to ensure that the book is flawless in terms of the grammar as well as its scientific presentation. Most important was his moral support to ensure that the book is completed on time and ready for publication.

PROLOGUE

A

"The greatest crisis facing us is crisis in the organization and accessibility of human knowledge. We own an enormous "encyclopedia" which isn't arranged alphabetically. Our "file cards" are spilled on the floor. The answers we want may be buried somewhere in the heap"

(Robert Heinlein)

B

"The person who finds the study of nutrition interesting, fascinating and challenging, will most likely enjoy better health; very likely live longer and might enjoy the mission of helping his neighbors do the same "

(John M. Ellis)

C

"To improve the nutritional values of the citizens of the country, nutritional education must precede increased food production. An increased production of vegetables, milk,meat and other products without having first raised demand for these products beforehand would result in the failure of the project".

(Anonymous)

D

''It is vitally important for employers to get involved in the diet patterns of their employees in order to make them healthy and fit. This ensures increased productivity by reducing absenteeism to almost zero on health grounds''.

(HLN Anderson)

PREFACE

THE JOURNEY OF LIFE

Modern civilization tries to solve the problem of death and birth by thinking in terms of possessions (progress and happiness) rather than the right way of living in terms of being or existence (harmony and wisdom).

People do not know how to nourish or heal themselves physically or spiritually. As a result, they lack energy for living and creativity. Most of them don't even know why they are in this world.

The secret of a serene, peaceful, happy and joyful life is being in harmony with the laws of nature – both physical and spiritual.

This includes knowing how to keep the physical body in harmony with nature as well as attaining spiritual harmony through living in accordance with God's rules. For a man or woman who strives to live by these two ideas, his or her eternity or heaven has already begun right here and now.

To be as healthy as possible, the wise man intervenes as little as possible. He lets things take their natural course. In the end, life always reasserts its right and wins every time.

Our over-technical and overspecialized medical system is based on a slight error of emphasis. The modern miracle worker or expert concentrates on the machine and disease rather than on the person; and tends to disregard the mind in the treatment of the body and vice versa, so that the eventual healing is often partial, unsatisfactory and sometimes not permanent.

Refreshingly, one simple but highly concentrated act may be enough to restore or maintain a person's health. Physical health and harmony with the laws of nature and the world around us are completely interdependent. What we have tried to do in this book therefore is to unravel this interdependency as simply as possible to enable the lay person access and optimize it for life-long health and vitality.

For maximum physical strength, power, endurance and intellectual vigour nothing is comparable with man's original diet of grains, fruits, nuts and vegetables.

It is gratifying for those who are 40 years and above to note that health or fitness is ageless! One can be fit and healthy at any age. Even at 100 years, one can still be fit and healthy. Everything depends on lifestyle choices. Good nutrition and an active life are two crucial choices one must make to remain healthy and fit. Other important lifestyle choices include adequate restful sleep, good stress management, drinking alcohol moderately (if at all), abstaining from smoking, wearing of seatbelts, good personal hygiene, regular medical checkups and good interpersonal relationship.

But fitness is not the same as health. Fitness only looks at the physical aspect of health but health encompasses more: physical, mental, spiritual and social wellbeing.

Some footballers appear physically fit but sometimes they have been seen to collapse and die on the field from undiagnosed illnesses. An armedrobber may be physically fit but cannot be said to be healthy because he is not impacting society positively.

Millions of people walking the streets are already dead and don't know it. For most of these people, the epitaph on their graves should read: "Died at thirty, buried at sixty"

Over 95% of people we see on the street cannot pass minimum physical fitness test but most would be considered healthybecause they are going about doing their normal duties that impact positively on society.

While it is true that most human beings want to have excellent health from day to day and from year to year "till death do us part", very few (less than 1%) actually take necessary steps to undertake the lifestyle changes that protect health.

Governments and health practitioners pay lip service to preventive medicine and spend less than 1% of their health budget and even less percentage of their time on primary prevention of diseases. More disturbing is the fact that even the health practitioners who should know better often confuse primary withsecondary prevention of disease. The majority of health practitioners, including some doctors, spend most of their time and money on secondary prevention of diseases by focusing on early detection of established disease doing tests like mammograms, blood chemistry and PSA tests but devote very little time and money to helping the populace understand nutritional and life style changes necessary for primary prevention of diseases before they take holdin the body in the first place. This is a most tragic irony of modern medical practice that needs to be addressed urgently in the training curricular and in the general population if we are to make any progress in our health indices, disease burden and health expenditure on individuals, communities and the country at large.

It was Dr. Ray D. Strand (MD) who said that''Nutritional Medicine is foreign to most physicians as well as the public''.He believes that you don't have to be a physician to practice primary prevention of diseases. Anybody can become proactive about primary prevention of disease through the adoption and practice of the principles set out in this book as you allow food tobe your medicine and your medicine food.

The idea of teaching preventive health through diet has been of a low priority in orthodox medical schools.Refreshingly,a number of medical schools across the world are waking up tothe realityof this all-important aspect of medicine.Diseases should be prevented long before they take hold in the body. People should be told what foods to eatand those to avoid thereby preserving health for as long as possible rather than wait until they have damaged their bodies with harmful eating-lifestyle associated choices.

For instance, the first WHO Global Studies Report on Non-communicable Diseases (NCD) has listed Nigeria and other developing countries as the worst hit with deaths surpassing those of communicable diseases. The situation has been described as an impending disaster for our society, and our economy. The NCD include among others, cardiovascular diseases, stroke and diabetes. The WHO report had said that the situation can be remedied simply by diligent implementation of existing measures and policies like strong anti-tobacco control, promotion of healthier lifestyle, physical activity, control of alcohol consumption and improving diet and nutrition education as well as improved agricultural practice that will lead to the production of health promoting food crops e.g. gardening and animal husbandry.

To compound issues, the healthcare systems of these countries have failed woefully with iatrogenic diseases ranking as one of the greatest killers. These are attributed to adulterated drugs, quackery, poor equipment, poor infrastructure and poor training.

Indeed there is no need for foreign assistance or foreign products to solve Africa's health problem. The solution lies within us all! The solution does not require rocket science either. The major problem is with the African (or Nigerian) diet which lacks variety from meal to meal or from day to day. The foods are most often over-cooked with specific reference to the practice of re-warming stew over many days or weeks. And most grievously, the diet lacks fruits and vegetables! The result is a population with poor average IQ, high incidence of child mortality, stunted growth leading to haggard syphilitic habitures with unpleasant physiques. Poor nutrition also reflects on fertility, memory, energy level, economic productivity and high maternal mortalityas well as increase in non-communicable diseases that is fast becoming one of the greatest causes of morbidity and mortality in these countries.

In view of the foregoing, a book like this one is timely and an imperative to tackle the huge burden of diseasesthat is very dismal vital statistical indices prevalent in the countries. The book is indeed a compendium of scientific evidence-based principles thatwill serve as a practical guide, personal mentor and reference on nutrition for individuals, health practitioners, communities and institutions to help, prevent and control both communicable and non-communicable diseases in the country.

I can therefore, happily recommend this well-written book to individuals, schools and institutions as a general studies guide to promote health and prevent and control diseases which have plagued our people and blighted our developmental efforts as a nation.

Dr. Thomas A. Affi.

CHAPTER 1
INTRODUCTION

The above axiom is true and correct today as it was in the days of Seneca centuries ago. The way you look, think and behave are the veritable result of what you munch or do not munch at your breakfast, lunch or dinner each day. Depending on what you eat and how much you eat it, food can make you go fat or slim; idiotic, irritable or alert; peaceful and in control of yourself. Indeed, what you consume each day contributes immeasurably towards determining your very survival and ultimate destiny.

Disease never comes without a cause. The way is usually prepared and the disease is invited in as a result of unwise disregard for the natural laws of feeding. It was Herbert George, who, in the 17th century, summarized this concept best when he said that, ''whatever was the father of a disease, an ill diet was the mother''.

The natural laws of feeding are commonplace but like the wise say, commonsense is not common. We often therefore, need to be reminded of the existence of these laws of nature and their powerful influence on our day-to-day survival.

The day a man ceases to breathe marks only but an end-point of a process started much earlier in life through unwise and wrongful selection of food at meal times. The damage that leads to the ultimate demise of a man or woman actually begins much earlier in life. In fact, the life-expectancy of a man is to a large extent the sum-total of what he has eaten or not eaten while he had the opportunity to do so. Moreover, the statement – that the worst instruments of suicide are the knife and fork that we use each day at the table – is very true. We do not indeed die, but kill ourselves, albeit, slowly over many years of faulty feeding.

The wrongful choice of food is largely a result of ignorance but sometimes it is due to sheer vainglory and utter disregard for one's health in the misguided whim to gratify momentary indulgence.

Since ignorance is the greatest cause of poor feeding habits, I have tried in this book to remind us of the rules and regulations which if properly observed can help us live life to the full as God intended it.

As mentioned in the preface, eating correctly does not necessarily mean one would live forever, or even live to be 100 years as there are various other causes of death which include accidents. But barring accidents and other causes of un-natural death, correct choice of food can guarantee a long, useful and productive life to the very end. Such life is devoid of irritating and often debilitating illnesses that characterise gluttonous and wanton life-styles. Correct eating habits assure a full life that is vivacious, sparkling right into a ripe old age – both physically and mentally.

There is no age limit for starting to eat right for life-long vitality. No matter how old, everyone benefits from adopting the right eating culture. The results are often immediate and dramatic within weeks or months. There are examples of people who were given up for early premature death at 50 years of age or so in view of their debilitating illnesses but who, on adopting the right eating culture, had gone on to live to be 90 years or more. Their lives were not only lengthened but became disease-free and sparkling right up to the very end.

It has become almost a cliché in my office when I tell my patients that old age is not synonymous with ill health. It is gratifying to know, particularly, for those who are 40 years and above, that health or fitness is ageless. One can be fit and healthy at any age.

Since ignorance is the greatest factor that militates against healthy eating habits, I have unapologetically devoted a large part of the book to educating the reader about the nutritional values of all the common foodstuffs available in the country. Such knowledge, I believe, is foundational and a prerequisite to changing one's long-established faulty habits. As someone aptly put it "Education is not about knowing more but about behaving differently".

For instance, it is a fact that by drinking a single bottle of soft drink, one consumes not less than seven cubes of white sugar. We also know that white sugar is singularly injurious to health. This creates awareness about the necessity to cut down on the number of bottles of soft drinks people take in a day. Another example will make this point even clearer. It is a known fact that excessive consumption of table salt predisposes some people to hypertension and its attendant destructive outcomes. We also know that certain foodstuffs contain unusually high amount of salt. Examples of high salt foods are bread, cheese, soft drinks, margarine, bacon and sardines. These two related facts go a long way to create awareness in wise people to cut down on these high salt foods. This is especially important for those who already have hypertension.

In addition to knowing the exact nutritional values of each food item one eats, it is equally important to know what quantity of each food one should eat at a sitting.

The general rule of thumb is to eat everything in moderation. The golden rule of eating right is to eat sparingly. Most people eat far too much for their own good, especially with respect to particular food items. The result is usually ill health and premature aging. In fact, if we all eat a quarter(¼) of what we eat in a day, our hospital beds will be virtually empty, most of the time.

The belief in our culture that being overweight or obese is a sign of good living is as fallacious as it is primitive. Nothing could be further from the truth. Obesity, if anything is a sign of one's gradual and painful departure from this world. Overweight people who have pot-bellies and fat necks are losing out on a full and enjoyable life. Each day of their life is troubled by frequent irritating and often debilitating illnesses. They may live long but their lives are empty and miserable. Such people may appear to be living glamorous lives but all that is skin-deep or indeed "fat-deep". For them, every little movement is a miserable effort, ranging from their daily wash to doing their routine work in the office. The only way to live life to the full is to maintain an ideal body weight that allows one to function optimally from minute-to-minute and from day to day. And the diet recommended in this book, buttressed by the breakthrough principle of eating according to blood type is guaranteed to help most people maintain their ideal body weight for maximum performance at work and at play right into a ripe old age.

Centuries of experience and experimentation have proved beyond reasonable doubt that eating sparingly ensures lifelong vitality and prolongs useful life. In fact some extremists, like some Tibetan hermits, believe that a single meal a day is enough to keep body and soul together. This may be indeed correct in principle but is likely to prove inadequate for most people in the long run. For instance, a single meal may likely fail to supply all the necessary nutrients the body needs over a period of time. Moreover, a single meal a day may prove socially unacceptable in contemporary social settings. Nevertheless, this degree of extremism undoubtedly underscores the fundamental principle of eating sparingly for life-long vitality.

One other very important principle of eating correctly is the idea of eating foodstuffs in their natural state as much as possible. Foods are best eaten when they are fresh and straight from the farms, with little or no processing. Food processing, despite the aesthetic appeal that it imparts to the finished products, tends to impoverish food nutritionally and leave them in the unhealthiest form. Moreover, processed foods usually have certain chemicals added called preservatives or colouring agents. Some of these chemicals are potentially harmful on the long term.

Closely related to the principle of eating food in their most natural form is the need to eat foods of plant origin and avoid animal foods as much as possible. I am not in any way suggesting strict vegetarianism or anything of the sort but all I am saying is that eating animal foods like red meat and dairy products in large quantities is detrimental to good health. This principle has a far reaching effect on our minute-to-minute, day-to-day quality of life as well as the long-term survival. Too much animal food is linked with shortened life-span and unhappy day-to-day living.

Anatomically, the human digestive system of man is not suited to flesh eating because man has flat teeth adapted to chewing of vegetable food compared to the sharp cutting teeth of carnivorous mammals. In addition, man's gut has a long intestinal tract that is more suited to vegetarian diet compared to the short intestines of meat-eating animals.

Even the scriptures initially did not support the eating of flesh by man. For instance when God created the first man and woman he had instructed them to eat only plant foods like grains, nuts, and seeds. And when man stuck to this God-decreed diet, his life-span had ranged from 600 – 969 years. Meat eating was only permitted to man as fallout of Noah's flood that destroyed most plant sources of food. And since then, man's life-span has reduced drastically from about 600 years to less than 200 years at the time of Abraham; and down to less than 120 years in our time.

Current scientific evidence is that despite the fact that much damage has been done over thousands of years of flesh-eating by our ancestors, we can improve considerably on our quality of life and life-span by simply cutting down on flesh-foods and reverting to the God-decreed diet of grains, seed, nuts, fruits and vegetables. This will improve our temperaments; give us clear minds, clear eyes and disease-free bodies for years on end.

For instance, science has proved that an adult person needs only 0.15 – 0.20g of protein per kg body-weight per day for health. This adds up to less than 5% of the total calorie a person needs to eat per kg per day. Pregnant women and growing children however, need a little more protein (about 0.6 – 0.9g per body weight per day). Any excess above these stated figures is as wasteful as it is harmful. Wasteful because the excess meat is passed in faeces and urine; harmful because animal products contain saturated fat which causes premature ageing of blood vessels, especially of the heart, leading to heart attack or heart failure. A high protein diet is one of the reasons why heart attacks and heart failure is now the commonest cause of death in industrialized countries. People in these countries eat excessive amount of animal foods such as meat, cheese, milk and milk products. This pattern is beginning to rear its ugly head here in developing countries like Nigeria especially amongst the more affluent members of our society who ignorantly abandon the much healthier African diet for unhealthy western food in the name of sophistication. To avoid this grievous mistake, we must begin to educate our young ones on the vital need to eat only fresh, unprocessed foods, preferably "straight from the farm".

Another major cause of faulty feeding is the unhealthy habits of letting our appetites dictate to us what we should eat or not eat. In the practice of healthy eating, the appetite is not the best guide to selecting what we should eat. Indeed, if we are to cultivate the habit of eating right, we must bear in mind the following utilitarian cliché which says that for optimum health "we must eat what we would rather not, and avoid that which we would rather eat".

Cardiovascular diseases are increasing towards epidemic proportions in developing countries as they already account for one-third (⅓) of global deaths and almost 10% of global burden of disease and are set to become the leading cause of deaths in the developing world very soon.

 If we are to cultivate the desirable habit of eating correctly for life-long day–to-day vitality, we must break the routine of allowing the clock to dictate what times we eat. Most of us eat because it is time for lunch or dinner without considering whether or not we are hungry. It is a most unhealthy habit indeed. What time we eat must be dictated by whether or not we are hungry enough to eat at that particular time. Hunger is a reliable, automatic, in-built mechanism within our body system which tells us when the body needs "refueling". When the hunger signal is not yet flashing it means that the system is happy with what it is working with, so that any unsolicited addition only goes to interfere with the smooth and effective functioning of the entire system and may even harm it in the long term.

If such "unsolicited" overloading of the system goes on unchecked day after day, month after month and year after year, the system is likely to break down and manifest as disease. Indeed, it would be desirable and healthy to allow ourselves to 'starve' a little between meals to ensure that previous food eaten is properly digested and thoroughly "burnt out" and the system is well cleaned out before the next batch of food is "loaded" in. This ensures maximum efficiency of the system. I personally have found this practice most gratifying and rewarding, both physically and mentally.

It is my firm belief that whoever reads this book and applies the principles enunciated therein to himself or herself, no matter how young or old, he or she will discover a whole new life full of vitality in all its ramifications.

I am by no means saying that applying the principles in this book will guarantee longevity. Most people are not even interested in living that long anyhow. What I do promise, however, and which is the desire of most men and women the world over, is a life that is productive and full of "joie de vivre" from minute to minute and from day to day. Such life is devoid of those irritating or even disabling diseases that often rob it of its very worthiness. As the Americans would say "if you are gonna strike out, you might as well strike out swinging".

A good diet and regular exercise permit a woman to keep an attractive face and figure into the ninth decade. Remember Sarah, the wife of Abraham in the Bible had no puffy eyes in the morning, no swollen ankles in the evening. For men, it means staying physically fit and being able to put in long hours of work and play without feeling tired.

In conclusion, medical research has shown that giving animals the basic minimum of food required to keep them alive resulted in their living to twice their life expectancy. The experiment has been tested on humans and it appears to protect the heart, circulatory system and brain against age-related diseases like Alzheimer's. The study went ahead to conclude that dietary calorie restriction including regular fasting extends life expectancy and protects the brain and cardiovascular system against age-related diseases like cancer, diabetes mellitus and Alzheimer's disease.

CHAPTER 2
SHARING THE AFRICAN EXPERIENCE

"Research indicates that the human life-span may be doubled or even tripled by proper dieting in accordance with blood group, eating food sparingly and sleeping 7 to 8 hours per night"

(Anonymous)

A healthy eating pattern and positive lifestyle changes are your best approaches to staying healthy and preventing disease or at least slowing down its course. The aim is to eat smartly to prevent and manage diseases throughout your life.

The choices you make about food each day, along with your physical activity, affect your health and how you feel today, tomorrow and in the future.

Your life is filled with choices. Every day you make thousands of choices many of which are related to food. Some seem trivial, others are important. But as insignificant as a single choice may seem, if it is made over and over again over many days, months and years, it can have a major or even catastrophic consequence for you and your family members.

The practical steps and flexible guidelines in this book will help you choose correctly nutritious foods to match your own individual needs, preferences and lifestyles in other to change your life for the better. Eating for health is one of the wisest decisions you will ever make.

This book fills this crucial gap in our knowledge of what we should eat for good health and what we should avoid in order to assure life-long vitality and health.

The primary aim of this book is not necessary to teach people how to live to be 100 years old, but to encourage individuals and families to live lives that are vivacious, productive and sparkling from minute-to-minute, from hour-to-hour and from day-to-day. What is the point of living to be 100 years when half of those years are spent in and out of hospitals? Or what is the point living to be 80 years but without one's sight, hearing or one's mental capacity? As I mentioned above, the aim is not to prevent death but help people die healthy.

There are already several good books on nutrition and health in the market, but this one hopes to take its unique place for the following reasons. Most books on nutrition in the market talk about foods and food practices of developed countries of Europe and America. This volume is however, concerned with African foods and practices relevant to our environment and culture. What I have done is to practically translate the abundant scientific research findings on nutrition and health into a language that the layman can read and understand. I have therefore tried to present these facts in simple readable Nigerian English. I have as much as possible tried to avoid controversial areas as well as intricate statistics of scientific research. For as I said elsewhere, one does not have to be a mechanical engineer to be able to drive a car well.

I must proclaim from the outset that most of the facts, assertions and recommendations in this book are by no means my original thoughts or discoveries. Nevertheless, before I put down these assertions, I have either tried them on myself or else I have cross-checked them thoroughly in the relevant current medical or nutritional literature to assure their authenticity.

I first became fascinated with the science of nutrition and health as far back as 1978 after we had completed the dissection of a human body during the first few years of medical school in Zaria. Having seen the in and out of the human body, I became intensely interested in how to preserve health and prevent disease in the human body. I soon became obsessed with the idea of health and vitality and thereupon embarked on extensive literature review on nutrition in particular and health in general.

I also began to apply the knowledge so acquired to myself to find out the truth about what I had read in the literature. I tried out a number of diets, for their effects on my physical as well as mental capacity. For instance, I used to go on fruits alone for a day or two to find out the effect on my health. It reached a point I stopped taking white sugar, based on the result of experiments carried out on myself. This was way back in 1978 when I was in my third year of medical school. I also avoided coffee from as far back as 1979.

I have persisted with this personal experimentation and literature review for the past 30 years or more. The result is the book you are now about to read.

In this book you will find a lot of recommendations against several established cultural and traditional food practices. Some of them are almost heretical as far as established cultural practices are concerned. Imagine telling Nigerians to cut down on palm oil, maize and palm wine. It is simply revolutionary.

It is my sincere hope that the secrets unfolded in this book will be made to reach all Africans in general and Nigerians as an individual fundamental human right to ensure long vitality and health. This can be achieved most expediently by teaching them at the secondary and tertiary levels of our educational system. It is incumbent on government to make it possible for every citizen to get to know how to take care of himself or herself in order to make them productive and useful to himself in particular and the nation in general.

Diet (Gk, diatia = mode of living) once referred to one's general way of life with regards to dressing, behavior, and mental attitude as a means of shaping one's destiny. Today the term is restricted to the food regime one follows. Although the idea that it is connected with one's fate is often implicated in it. The best food is said to be that which is grown or cultivated in one's own country; and for each season the fruits and vegetables of that season are the best. The true native should therefore eat the produce of his native soil. The more a person partakes of foreign foods the more he is said to lose his native disposition and natural wisdom. Modern work has shown that persons who change their native diet to alien ones are more prone to hypertension and other nutritional diseases: obesity, heart and other disease conditions like mental sluggishness. Seneca (A.D. 65), said, "More people are killed through the stomach than by the sword".

The information in this book is very much in line with Federal Government philosophy of education which is to impart relevant educational material that will remain with the student long after he or she leaves school, in order for him or her to be useful to himself or herself in particular and the society in general for the rest of his of her life. It is true, the saying that, "education is what is left after one may have forgotten all he/she learnt in school."

I entirely agree with Mr. Pekka Puska (now Professor World Health Foundation) who summed up the topic most beautifully as follows: "People can choose wisely only if well informed. In today's world information on risk factors and healthy choices should be a fundamental human right. It is a major responsibility of governments to ensure that the people are knowledgeable about these matters. Particular attention should be given to young children and adolescents in schools. It is as important to learn how to stay healthy as it is to study academic subjects".

In order to achieve the above objective, the book apart from being a must for all family libraries, should be recommended text for Senior Secondary Schools, Schools of Nursing and Midwifery, School of Health and Technology, Medical Schools and undergraduates in their first year of University education as part of their General Studies curriculum.

The book is not the compilation of one man or any one person's original idea but a compendium of facts and figures gleaned over the past 30 years from researchers and scholars all over the world and from all generations for the benefit of our people and children yet unborn. What I have done essentially is to domesticate, repackage and communicate the nutritional information from an African perspective for local consumption, digestion and assimilation. Talk of thinking global and acting local, for the benefit of our citizenry.

HISTORICAL PERSPECTIVE

Colonization of Africa by Europeans brought along with it a poor western diet that has been inadvertently copied by native Africans as status symbol and hallmark of sophistication with the attendant serious consequence of a wide range of diseases which had hitherto been unknown in Africa. The colonial western diet consisted of the following:

1. Diet based on processed white flour and white sugar (white bread, pastries, cakes, doughnuts, chin-chin, meat pie)
2. Animal fats (pork, fat, butter, margarine, trans-fats, lard)
3. Well-peeled or fried potatoes
4. Salt and spices in abundance (pickles, steaks and sauces)
5. Desserts/sweets loaded with white sugar.

Fresh vegetables and fruits were scarce, as they were not considered nutritionally important. And to make matters worse addiction to a number of toxic stimulants (coffee, tobacco, alcohol and other drugs) was considered attractive and a sign of liberation or social arrival.

From the beginning of the 2nd half of the twentieth century, science began to link some of the prevailing diseases to such impoverished diet; especially to dietary deficiencies.

The message is that if people adopt life-styles that are health promoting and disease preventing then their health care cost and expenditures, both national and individual, would be drastically reduced. This is the quintessence of the primary health care programme which has been adopted by Governments all over the world in response to the Alma Ata Declaration of 1978.

The most important fact of health promotion and disease prevention has to do with what people eat or do not eat. This in turn depends very much on the levels of awareness as to what is nutritionally good and what is not so good for the body.

CULTURAL PERSPECTIVE

From the cultural perspective, the African or Nigerian diet is seriously flawed in several respects as follows:

1. Timing of meals

Most Nigerians and indeed most Africans don't have respect for time, hence the unfortunate aphorism of "African time"! Africans and particularly Nigerians may claim to eat 3 square meals a day but the exact time is of no consequence to them. Breakfast time for instance, can be anything from 7.00 am and to 11.00 am. This range can further vary from day to day or week to week. The person takes breakfast at 8.00 am today and depending on his or her events and temperament, breakfast could be postponed till about 10.30 am or 11.00 am the next day. But science has shown that fixed meal times go a long way to allow food consumed to be properly digested, absorbed and assimilated.

Therefore, as explained later in the book, the time variation for a particular meal should not exceed one hour. For instance, breakfast should vary between 7.00 am – 8.00 am and not more; and time variation for lunch should not go beyond one hour, which is between 1.00 pm and 2.00 pm. Similarly the best time range for dinner should be one hour; from 6.30 pm to 7.30 pm.

2. Deep Frying

According to Dr. Joel Wallack, the deep frying of foods, with particular reference to fast foods, is responsible for a large percentage of non-communicable diseases that plague the modern man including cancer, arthritis, coronary heart disease, stroke, hypertension or even diabetes mellitus. The process of frying converts fats or oils into harmful toxins especially trans-fats. The worst aspect is that the fumes given off during deep frying is particularly injurious to the person cooking especially women who do the cooking. They are seriously exposed to the risk of cancers of the breast and ovaries from these fumes.

A related and culturally harmful practice is the reheating of Nigerian "stews". Some families reheat a particular pot of stew for well over 3 days, one week or even one month. This most deleterious practice must be abandoned nationally in all families. We must revert to the healthier ancestral practice of cooking soup and eating the whole lot over one meal and wash the pot against the next day. This practice had immeasurably contributed to the legendary longevity of our ancestors who lived long and had retained their five senses and thinking faculties into ripe old age!

3. Abandoning of Local Seasoning Agents

Before the arrival of the colonial masters, Africans and Nigerians in particular had used their local traditional seasoning agents like locust beans, soya beans and others. But with the coming of colonialism, these healthy seasoning agents were abandoned for harmful seasonings like MSG. The clarion call now is for all families to return to using African local and traditional seasoning agents to ensure health and longevity.

4. Lack of Fruits/Vegetables in Our Local Diets

A cursory observation validates this Achille's heel of the African and (in particular) the Nigerian diet. Most families eat little or no fruits and vegetables. They consume fruits only once in a long while when it is available in season or is given them free. Vegetables are usually restricted to overcooked green leaves in soups used to garnish rice, yam or potato.

The WHO recommends that at least 400g per day of fruits and vegetables (including 30g/day from pulse, nuts and seeds). But the African and particularly the Nigerian actual intake range from 60 – 160g/day (very poor indeed). This severe lack of fresh raw fruits and vegetables may very well indeed explain the very short life-expectancy of Nigerians and Africans in general compared to countries like Japan, Israel and China where their life-expectancy nearly doubles ours. Government must therefore do more to promote the cultivation of fruits and vegetables nationally as well educate citizens to eat same through publications such as this one and other media.

5. Large Dinners

Our ancestral practice of eating little or nothing in the morning and something small in the afternoon, only to swallow large meals at supper is to say the least, topsy–turvy nutritionally. Eating large meals at dinner interferes with sleep, promotes obesity and has far reaching consequences on the kidneys and the liver. No wonder the incidence and prevalence of kidney and liver failures are rampant across the country. The largest and the most nutritious meal of the day should be breakfast and not supper. The last meal of the day – supper – should be decidedly small and very light. This allows the person to sleep peacefully through the recommended seven to eight hours at night without disruption.

6. Culture of Dead Foods

Another serious fault with the diet of fellow Nigerians is the culture of eating cooked and boiled foods at breakfast, lunch and dinner with little or no fresh foods throughout the day, throughout the week and for months on end. Cooked foods are literally dead foods that cannot be expected to produce anything but dead or half-dead people. That is why some people feel that some Nigerians walking around are virtually dead by 30 years of age and only get buried at 60.

A recent survey of the health of Nigerians showed that by the age of 45 years, nearly half of the citizens are battling one or more chronic diseases that make them function like one-cylinder cars. For good health and longevity, therefore, every citizen should eat at least 50% of his food raw or half cooked. This will go a long way to protect us against life-blighting and life-shortening diseases. Hence the need to focus on fruit and vegetable production in the country.

7. The Extremes of Red Meat Consumption

There is the funny paradigm in the African or Nigerian pattern of red meat consumption that is highly inimical to health and longevity. The paradox is that those who have access to red meat eat it to excess and those who have little or no access to red meat go without it virtually all year round from one Christmas or Sallah to another. Both practices are inimical to long healthy life.

The consumers of excess red meat tend to suffer from chronic non-communicable diseases like diabetes, cancer and arthritis. While those who eat little or no red meat are often protein–calorie deficient and tend to suffer and die prematurely from communicable infectious diseases because of lowered immunity.

8. Patronage of Junk Foods

In a house where the father and mother are working outside the home, it is almost impossible for them to prepare home produced meals that require time and more effort to prepare. This is especially so if there are children to be prepared and sent off to school. The options available to working couples are junk foods (tea and bread, couscous or indomie), or overcooked left over dead foods that are heated over and over again. Both options are equally harmful.

Recommendations:

1. Wife is to cook in the evenings, prepare and pack in good warmers against morning.
2. Patronize mama put bukas for home grown rather than fast food.
3. Women should become fulltime housewives till children are out of school.
4. Employ local cooks who can cook healthful local meals in the house while husband and wife are off to work.
5. Combination of two or more of the above options.

CHAPTER 3

WHY THE SUDDEN EMPHASIS ON FOOD AS MEDICINE?

"The longer I live, the less confidence I have in drugs and the greater is my confidence in the regulation and administration of diet and regimen"

John Redman Coxe

According to a report of the Nutrition Institute of America (NIA) in 2003, the number one cause of death in the United States of America, the world's leading nation in healthcare spending, as well as health research, development and technology, is attributed to iatrogenic causes followed by heart diseases as number two and cancer as number three.

Cause	Number of Patients
Iatrogenic	784,000
Heart Diseases	699,692
Cancer	553,251

(Iatrogenic = Caused by doctors, therapist, pharmacist, nurses, etc).

The following are some of the factors that contribute to the high incidence of iatrogenic diseases:

a.   Mistakes in treatment

b.   Errors in surgery

c.   Medical errors

d.   Wrong drugs

e.   Wrong diagnosis

f.   Radiation from x-ray

g.   Negligence

h.   Delayed treatment

The above informs the imperative for renewed emphasis on primary prevention of disease through appropriate food selection and consumption.

A similar study was undertaken in Australia many years ago to determine the impact of iatrogenic diseases in that country's vital indices. It was discovered that iatrogenic diseases came 2nd as the commonest cause of mortality in that country. Although, I am not aware of any similar study in Nigeria, or indeed in Africa, but your guess would be as good as mine that the situation could be worse compared to that of America or Australia.

It was in this same light that Navarro the great Latino writer wrote in one of his books that the whole world would be a lot healthier without health workers. He said people are negligent about their health because they believe that doctors and other health workers are there to take care of them. They therefore refuse to accept that primary prevention of disease is far better than treatment. It is wiser and more economical to take responsibility for one's health to prevent disease from taking a foothold in one's body in the first place than wait till one has the disease then go for early diagnosis and treatment.

Except for unforeseeable accidents and with a few very exceptional cases, most diseases can be prevented primarily before they take hold in our bodies if we take the trouble to eat correctly and effect some lifestyle changes for health.

This is the major thrust of this book in that it is a pragmatic guide to primary prevention of disease; a compendium of relevant principles for maintaining good health into ripe old age instead of building more hospitals.

CHAPTER 4
HOW WOULD YOU KNOW YOU ARE HEALTHY?

"A sad soul can kill you quicker than germs"
(John Steinbeck)

Wellness is a relatively recent concept. Health or wellness means more than physical health. A healthy person is one who is physically healthy and in addition exists in a dynamic involving relationship with his or her environment including emotional, intellectual, spiritual, social and physical environment. In other words, there are six interrelated dimensions of health that need to be in place for one to be said to be fully alive and vibrant:

1. **Physical Wellness:** To be physically healthy, one needs to take charge of the following: diet, exercise, avoid harmful habits like drugs and substance abuse, engage in sex responsibly and take time to do annual medical check-ups as at when due. This includes regular immunization for children and adults.

2. **Emotional Health:** this requires that a person be responsible enough to be trustworthy, have self-confidence and maturity in dealing with other people. The person should be bold enough to share his or her feelings with confidants and other significant people in his or her life. An emotionally healthy person puts other people before him or herself. In other words, the person is not hedonistic but stoic, compassionate and empathetic.

3. **Intellectual Wellness:** this requires that one keeps an open mind and tolerates other people's views and opinions without been overly critical. The person is very understanding and accommodating but retains the capacity to be curious and to question injustice and oppression. He/she also retains the ability to laugh at himself when necessary and displays a good sense of humour and creativity when in the midst of others.

4. **Spiritual Wellness:** this means that a person lives by a set of principles and beliefs that inherently give him positive meaning and purpose for living. The best example is commitment to organized religion of some sort that gives capacity for the practitioner to be compassionate, merciful, forgiving and altruistic.

5. **Social Wellness:** this refers to having and enjoying satisfying relationship that are fulfilling and non-manipulative. To achieve this level of wellness

and health, one needs to learn to practice good communication skills with special reference to learning to be a good listener.

6. **Environmental Wellness:** in other to be fully healthy, it is important that the person takes the responsibility to be in harmony with his or her physical environment in order to ward off environmental pollution and animal violence. Wellness requires that one learns and protects him or herself against such hazards and doing one's best to control or eliminate these hazards as set out in this book.

The goodnews of this book is people have some control over whether they develop heart disease, cancer and other chronic diseases by the choices they make every day. Our job and that of the government is to provide the information, advice and encouragement but it is totally up to the individual to heed and live well or do otherwise and suffer.

Most people who are breaking all the health rules and principles do so because they don't know any better. They don't even know their current habits and lifestyles are harmful. Students who go about eating junk foods and sleeping poorly, drinking alcohol and getting involved in illicit sex may not know that they are harming themselves.

Herein lies the very crucial role of government to make it mandatory for all citizens to be educated in relation to what habits and lifestyles are good and which ones are harmful. The health education should begin very early from primary to secondary and into the tertiary institutions.

The health education should include relevant topics and issues as well as what resources are available to help one change behavior. Equally important is the knowledge about the person and how he relates to the wellness profile and also how to improve on each specific variable.

It is much easier to know when you are sick than when you are healthy because signs of good health are usually more subtle and vague. However, a healthy person is usually free from frequent attacks of infections like coughs, catarrh, fever or headaches. He or she does not get tired easily but performs his/her daily social and economic responsibilities feeling happy and energetic. To test your fitness you don't necessarily have to run 100 yards in 9 seconds or do 100 push-ups in one minute! All that is required for health is the absence of obvious disease and the ability of the individual to carry on his or her daily chores, work and play without hindrance. On the physical level, if a person can climb a set of stairs without difficulty, or walk a mile in 15 minutes, he or she is considered fit.

VITAL SIGNS OF HEALTH

Vital signs include blood pressure, pulse rate, respiratory rate and body temperature. A resting pulse rate of between 50 – 80 beats/minute taken on waking in the morning before you leave bed is considered within normal range. A resting respiratory rate of between 12–18 cycles per minute is normal. Normal body temperature taken on waking in the morning ranges from $35.2 – 37.2^0C$.

Blood pressure of 120/80 or lower is normal.

Using the vital signs and a few additional parameters of health, we can actually grade our health in order to guide us in an effort to improve our health. By applying appropriate lifestyle changes, one can actually move up from grade D to grade A^+ within.

In particular, a rising or high pulse rate is a very ominous sign that points to premature death.

Dr. Affi's Health Grading for Adults 18 years and above

S/N	Parameter	A^+	A	B	C	D
1	Pulse rate	50 – 59	60 – 64	65 – 69	70 – 74	75 – 80
2	BP (Systolic)	90 – 99	100 – 109	110 – 119	120 – 129	130 – 139
3	BP (Diastolic)	50 – 59	60 – 69	70 – 79	80 – 89	90 – 95
4	FBG	3.0 – 3.4	3.5 – 3.9	4.0 – 4.4	4.5 – 4.9	5.0 – 5.6
5	Hb	16.9 – 16.0	15.9 – 15.0	14.9 – 14.0	13.9 – 13.0	12.9 – 12.0
6	Respiratory Rate	12 – 14	15 – 17	18 – 20	21 – 23	24
7	Body Temperature	37.2	37.0	36.8	36.6	36.4
8	Cholesterol (total)	4.0	4.5	5	6	6.5
9	BMI	18 – 19	20 – 21	22 – 23	24 – 25	26 – 27
10	Sleep (Hours)	8	7	6	5	4

Score: $A^+ = 5$; $A = 4$; $B = 3$; $C = 2$; $D = 1$

$$\frac{TOTAL}{50} \times 100$$

Range: 20 – 100%

BOWEL OPENING: Bowel opening is a veritable parameter for measuring wellness. The number of bowel openings per day, stool consistency and colour are very useful indicators of health.

Although the exact number of bowel openings per day or per week varies from individual to individual, the number remains constant for the person and any change should alert the person to the possibility of ill-health.

A good stool should be firm, soft, and torpedo-shaped and passed without difficulty. Any change from this calls for prompt check up. The colour of stool usually reflects the colour of food eaten but it should never be grey or very pale, very dark or bright red. Any of these colours call for immediate investigation.

URINE: Normal urine colour should be clear to pale amber. This colour generally indicates proper functioning of the liver and absence of urinary tract disease infection or cancer.

TONGUE APEARANCE: While the eye is the window of the soul, the tongue is the window to the body. For a person that is healthy, his tongue looks wet and is of pinkish colour without any fur but with visible papillae all over. A pale, or red smooth tongue with or without furring calls for prompt investigation.

The tongue of a healthy person that is well nourished and with adequate minerals and vitamins should have the following characteristics:

a.   Moderate in size (not too small not too big).

b.   Pink in colour all over evenly.

c.   Edges should be smooth and without teeth marks or indentation.

d.   There should be no coating or furring of any sort

e.   Taste buds or papilla should uniformly cover the surface and edges of the tongue.

f.   Wet

HOW WOULD YOU KNOW YOU ARE NOT HEALTHY?

The World Health Organisation defines health as the complete physical, mental and social well-being and not just the absence of disease. The following lists are harbingers and indicators of ill-health which must be taken seriously if we are to enjoy life-long health and vitality.

THE HARBINGERS OF ILL-HEALTH

S/N	Harbinger
1	Age over 40 years
2	High blood pressure
3	Diabetes mellitus
4	Stress
5	Overweight
6	Family history of heart disease
7	Smoking
8	Arterial disease
9	Stroke
10	Kidney disease
11	Gender
12	Sedentary lifestyle
13	Hyperlipidaemia

WARNING SYMPTOMS OF ILL-HEALTH

Physical

S/N	Symptom
1	Headaches (persistent)
2	Tightness around shoulder and neck
3	Abdominal pains
4	Constipation
5	Back pain
6	Sweaty palms
7	Dizziness
8	Sleep difficulties
9	Restless legs syndrome

10	Tiredness (unusual)
11	Ringing in ears

Behavioural

S/N	Symptom
1	Overuse of alcohol
2	Compulsive eating
3	Inability to get things done
4	Bossiness
5	Smoking
6	Bruxism (teeth grinding)
7	Critical and judgmental

Emotional Symptoms

S/N	Symptom
1	Crying easily
2	Nervousness
3	Anxiety
4	Boredom
5	Edgy – ready to explode any moment
6	Feeling powerless to change things
7	Overhauling sense of pressure
8	Anger
9	Lankiness
10	Unhappiness for no reason
11	Easily upset

Spiritual Symptoms

S/N	Symptom
1	Emptiness – no meaning to life
2	Prayerlessness
3	Doubt oneself
4	Lack of self confidence
5	Martyrdom

6	Looking for miracles to solve life's problem
7	Loss of direction
8	Cynicism
9	Apathy
10	Needing to prove oneself

Mental Symptoms

S/N	Symptom
1	Trouble concentrating
2	Forgetfulness
3	Lack of creativity
4	Memory loss
5	Inability to make decisions
6	Constant worry
7	Loss of sense of humour

Relational Symptoms

S/N	Symptom
1	Isolation
2	Intolerance
3	Resentment/unforgiving
4	Lashing out
5	Hiding from occasions/people
6	Lowered sex drive
7	Nagging
8	Distrust
9	Lack of intimacy
10	Manipulative
11	Few contacts with friends and relations

CHAPTER 5
HOW WOULD YOU KNOW YOU NEED DETOXIFICATION?

"Man so rich in knowledge has also become rich in diseases, but poor in health and physical strength"

(Sebastian Kneipp)

The irony of modern life is that even though we have so many machines and gadgets to make our lives 10 times easier than our ancestors, who lived just a few decades ago, yet we often wake up feeling more tired and sleepy than they felt. We are over-worked, overstressed, overfed and yet malnourished. This is so because throughout the history of mankind on earth, the present generation is living in the most polluted and toxic environment ever. The pollution is man-made through food, air, water and things that we come in contact with at home, work and play. Pollutants or toxins are substances that enter our bodies which are not nutrients and which are harmful when they accumulate in our bodies over time. Some can actually kill instantly if they enter the body in enough quantity e.g. Arsenic, carbon monoxide, lead and mercury.

The common pollutants and toxins in our environment include heavy metals, hormones, pesticides, insecticides, herbicides, antibiotics, plastic chemicals (PCB, BPA), food additives, food preservatives, drugs, air-fresheners, cosmetics, hydrogenated fats, dairy products, caffeine, etc.

Common sources of pollutants and toxins

1.	Caffeine in beverages and soft drinks

2.	Animal (agricultural) products

(a)	Meat products: They may contain pesticides, herbicides, insecticides and hormones.

(b)	Packaged meat, cured (smoked) meat and processed meat contain nitrates which may form cancer-causing nitrosamines.

(c)	Grilled meat (suya, balongu, kilishi)- the grilling process converts the oils and fats to pollutants.

3.	Trans-fats in commercial oils, margarine, fast foods, and fried foods generally. They are found in most breads and almost all baked foods, snacks, and fast foods and are linked to cancers, heart disease and stroke.

4.	Food additives - e.g. aspartame or nutrasweet is linked to memory loss, fatigue, dizziness, nausea, blurred vision, depression, hypersensivity reaction in children and ringing in the ear.

35

5.   Drugs/Medicines: some patients are often placed on 5 – 7 drugs at a time. Their side effects and interactions lead to toxicity.

6.   Fruits/Vegetables: these may contain residual pesticides, herbicides   or insecticides. Fruits that have thick peels are safer e.g. Oranges, grapefruit, banana. Fruit/vegetables that have thin peels (carrots, apple, broccoli, grapes, strawberries) are often loaded with toxins from the farm and thereafter. These thin-skinned fruits and vegetables need to be washed thoroughly before they are eaten. Washing with "exotic" detergents will remove virtually all toxins but even normal detergents and vinegar will do just as well.

Other sources of pollutants include:

7.	Penter ware	16.	Perfumes
8.	Paints	17.	Deodorants
9.	Glazed earthenware	18	Body Lotion
10.	Candle wick	19.	Dry Cleaning agent
11.	Hair dyes	20.	Newly painted house
12.	Canned food	21.	New carpet/furniture
13.	Ceramic dishes/cups	22.	Car exhaust
14.	Sea foods – Fish		
15.	Pesticides		

SIGNS AND SYMPTOMS OF TOXICITY: (MULTIPLE CHEMICAL SENSITIVITY)

If you have any of the following symptoms or signs for which common medical examination and tests fail to unravel any obvious cause, then you may well be suffering from one form of toxicity or the other. Efforts should be made to find the cause of the toxicity and at the same time, early detoxification is crucial. The common signs and symptoms of toxicity include:

1	Pimples	24	Mental symptoms
2	Recurrent boils	25	White-furred tongue that is difficult to brush off in the morning
3	Discolouration of the skin	26	Discolouration of teeth and gum
4	Jaundice	27	Lead taste in the mouth
5	Frequent headaches	28	Lead Jaundice (both eyes and skin stained

			earthy yellow)
6	Drowsiness	29	Lead emaciation (severe weight loss resembling HIV/ADS) but HIV negative
7	Wrinkles	30	Blue line along the teeth/gum junction
8	Premature aging	31	Loss of nail lunular
9	Grey hair (premature)	32	Fine tremors affecting handwriting
10	Poor vision	33	Unexplained nausea
11	Joint pains/stiffness	34	Unexplained renal disease
12	Persistent indigestion	35	Recurrent mouth ulcers
13	Muscle pains(non-specific)	36	Disorientation
14	General body pains	37	Panic attacks
15	Lack of sweating (even during exercise)	38	Palpitation
16	Paraesthesia	39	Unexplained tachycardia
17	Paralysis	40	Fluid in Lungs
18	Allergic reaction	41	Rashes
19	Chronic fatigue syndrome	42	Seizure disorder
20	Excessive sleepiness	43	Bloating
21	Arthritis	44	Shortness of breath
22	Forgetfulness		
23	Sugary taste		

HOW TO DETOXIFY FOR HEALTH

To detoxify effectively, first one must take the following steps to prevent toxins reaching one's body in the first place:

1. Eating according to blood group.
2. Avoid added a caffeine, tobacco, soft drinks, alcohol and fast foods.
3. Eat only organic foods if possible
4. Wash fruits and vegetables thoroughly with detergents or vinegar before eating
5. Do fruit fast: use the first 3 days of every month for convenience
6. Yoga exercise

7.   Sauna baths

8.   Aerobic exercise to sweat out toxins

9.   Expose body to sunlight for 10 to 20minutes a day (any time between 7:30am – 10:30am)

The main organ in the body that is involved in removing toxins from the body is the liver (90%). Other organs include the skin, the gut, the lungs and the kidneys. The following detoxifiers assist the liver to carry out its detoxification efficiently on a day to day basis.

Milk Thistle: This is also called Silymarin. It protects the liver and even stimulates it to produce new liver cells. Taking 200mg daily for 9 months resolves hepatitis and 175mg daily prevents any harming of the liver. It is also very beneficial in cancer of the liver and cirrhosis: It has to be taken for 8 weeks before it starts to show results.

Others include:

S/N	ITEM	S/N	ITEM
1	Spinach: eat daily (DABS)	22	Oats (dinner)
2	Broccoli (wash thoroughly first)	23	Noni drink
3	Cabbage	24	Sesame seeds
4	Green tea – blocks toxins (92%) from entering the body through food eaten from reaching the liver	25	Pumpkin seeds
5	Turmeric – Effects are similar to those of milk thistle.	26	Probiotics (dates and onion) – very useful during fasting period.
6	Strawberries	27	Fasting (fruit-fast for first 3days of every month and every Sabbath day)
7	Grapes/Grape seeds extracts	28	Multivitamin and multi-mineral supplement(Reload 50+)
8	Vitamin B12 injection-100mcg once a month for life	29	Tree nuts (Walnuts, Almonds, Cashew Nuts)
9	Chlorophyll supplement	30	Trevo cod liver oil
10	Spirulina	31	Peppermint

11	Zinc 15mg daily	32	Brewer's yeast – contains vitamin B_{15} an anti – dote to virtually all sorts of toxins
12	Cordyceps	33	Bitter leaf – prevents cancer from growing in liver (alfa – fetoprotein)
13	Garlic	34	Flax oil
14	Bitter kola	35	N-acetyl cysteine
15	Water drinking	36	Gamma oryzanol
16	Yoghurt	37	L- Glucosamine
17	L-Glutamine	38	Doxycycline
18	Coconut milk/ powder – treats prostate cancer	39	Curcumin 2000 – ease constipation in the elderly
19	Ginger – lowers blood sugar; Lowers BP in hypertension	40	Cinnamon – cures diabetes; protects the kidney
20	Rosemary	41	Sage tea
21	Cayenne pepper (added to green tea)		

Fasting for Detoxification

Fasting is one of the best ways to detoxify one's body. To detox properly and rapidly, one should use 3 days fruit juice fast rather than plain water fasting. One should restrict the fast to 3 days only. No need going for more that 3 days. The three days fruit juice fast may be repeated once every month continously. Using grapefruit juice is considered the gold standard but the juice of the following would do just as well depending on blood groups.

a.   Carrot juice

b.   Tomato juice

c.   Apple juice

d.   Beetroot juice

e.   Lemon juice

During the fast one should drink 300ml of the selected juice every 3hours. If it is not convenient to fast for 3days at a time, the next option is to use fruit juice fast on the Lord's rest day of Sabbath (Saturday) to coincide with Sabbath day i.e. fasting once a week for 52 weeks in a year (Compared to 3-day fast for twelve months in a year; totaling 36 fasting days). They however, can be done together i.e 1st 3 days of every month and then add every Sabbath day throughout the year.

In addition to detoxifying the body, fasting helps in healing most illnesses that plague man. Fasting can also cure addictions and substance abuse. Fasting literally changes things positively. This is because years of accumulated toxins in our bodies can make us live compromised, unfocused and unhealthy lives with no discipline. Fasting makes all that to fall away and frees the heart-dream you were born with and gives you refreshing vision and health.

Fasting changes a person to become more friendly, kind, joyful and peaceful. It is indeed a little death – a powerful tool given to you by God to slow down you fast-paced life and help you see where you are going and where you are coming from.

It also helps you to re-examine your values especially if there have been wasted years or meaningless pursuits.

It is indeed a pilgrimage to the desert of your soul where you will meet your greatest foe: your own weaknesses and there discover your strengths.

Fasting actually lifts us up above animal instincts and releases us from the cage of empty routines to unleash the creativity of a freed will. Fasting bestows on us such a beautiful countenance that makes us attractive and noble to behold. Fasting, when done correctly, and for a reasonable period (e.g. 3 days on grapefruit or orange juice) confers mental stability and often heals mental stress completely in certain cases. Finally, fasting helps us to be decisive, powerful, self-controlled and free. In short, fasting helps us to become the best we can be for God and man!!

CHAPTER 6
EATING ACCORDING TO BLOOD GROUP

After having successfully treated more than five hundred patients over the past five years based on the science of eating according to blood groups and food compatibility, I am thoroughly convinced beyond doubt that the efforts of pioneer workers in this field including Dr. James D'Adamo and his son, Dr. Peter J. D' Adamo, represent one of the greatest contributions to human progress and health, for which they deserve to be duly recognized and re-awarded. For it is indeed a medical breakthrough of all ages. This is because, eating according to blood group is seminal and fundamental to the promotion of health and the prevention and control of disease.

Each blood group contains genetic messages from our ancestors which affects us as individuals today. Knowing this predisposition helps us to understand the logic behind blood group versus food analysis concept.

A person's blood group determines the health, longevity, physical and emotional makeup of a person. Blood group and food analysis can make a difference between illness and health.

When you use your blood group as a guide for eating, you will be healthier; you will lose weight effortlessly and slow down the ageing process or even reverse it.

The blood group-food analysis has debunked forever the "one-diet-fit all" paradigm that have been wrongly propounded for centuries until very recently when the blood group breakthrough debuted in the late nineties.

The blood group diet works because it is based on scientifically proven cellular profile based on the food reactions in the person's body.

Foods are further grouped into 3 major categories: 'highly beneficial', 'neutral' and 'completely avoid'. The highly beneficial are foods that act like medicine when inside the person's body. The neutral group are foods that act like food; completely avoid refers to foods that act like poison when inside the body.

The diet has a very large variety of foods so that one does not have to worry about unnecessary rigid restrictions. The only requirement or prerequisite is for the individual to demonstrate preference for highly beneficial foods over the neutral foods but at the same time feel free to enjoy the neutral foods once in a while since they will not harm the person and in any case they contain nutrients that may be necessary for creating an adequate diet.

The secret therefore to balanced nutrition on this diet is to vigorously eliminate foods on 'completely avoid' list but eat those on the 'neutral list' except for the few that you personally feel might increase your body weight.

Any consideration for disease prevention and treatment should necessarily begin with blood group and food compatibility analysis.

In primary prevention of disease, blood group consideration should come first. So also in the treatment of disease; whether it is cancerous, infectious, nutritional, non-communicable or degenerative disease, one cannot succeed fully and completely in treating the condition without doing blood-food compatibility analysis. For standard medical practice, therefore blood and food analysis must precede all preventive and therapeutic interventions for total success.

Even today, some of my colleagues taunt me for placing so much emphasis on blood-food analysis in the treatment of patients. But I tell them that they are doing their best with what they know, but we are succeeding with what they don't know. In this regard, I fully agree with the saying that: unless the doctors of today choose to study and apply the science of nutrition to the treatment of patients, the dietitian of today will become the doctor of tomorrow.

The information about blood type and food analysis and its health implication is not rocket science. It is very simple and can be learnt and applied by doctors, nurses, family members and any interested person to maintain optimal health. I believe one does not have to be an automobile engineer to drive a car well. Therefore, I have deliberately avoided the scientific discourse on blood-food analysis. Instead, I have summarized the major aspects of their application in the tables for the sake of simplicity and across-board utility for the four blood groups. (See Appendix)

Though, the very last people to be convinced of any medical breakthrough are members of my constituency the medical doctors, yet considering the extreme potentiality of the practice of blood-food analysis, I urge and exhort my collegial faculty members to keep an open mind and embrace the practice for the sake of our suffering masses – the patients. A trial will convince even the most inveterate cynic that blood-food analyses is truly a fundamental medical breakthrough for all ages.

I equate it to a situation where two drugs are being compared in a double blind controlled trial in which one of the drugs is so good that you cannot help but stop the trial midway to enable the other patients also benefit.

CHAPTER 7
FASTING FOR HEALTH

Scientific studies and clinical results both corroborate the preventive and regenerative effects of fasting. Fasting, even for just once a month is said to cut the risk of coronary heart disease by 40%. The explanation is that fasting helps the body to rest from its metabolism, thereby enabling it to work more efficiently. The Sabbath one day fast is usually for 24 hours i.e. from six (6) pm on Friday to six (6) pm on Saturday the next day. The effect of fasting on coronary artery disease was seen to be true for diabetics as well, although they need to fast under the supervision of their doctor.

For effective healing however, the fast should last a minimum of 7 days and not more than 10 days without doctor's supervision.

HOW FASTING HEALS

Fasting has been associated with promoting health as well as curing certain illnesses such as cancer, immune diseases, addictions and some inflammatory conditions. During a fast, the white blood cells called lymphocytes, seek out toxins in the body and destroy them. This leaves the body cleaner and more energetic to facilitate healing. When one is fasting, the activities of digestion and absorption which normally take up two-thirds (2/3) of the body's energy is suspended leaving adequate energy available for healing process to take place, because the process of healing, since creation, is energy-intensive.

JUICE FASTING

From accumulated experience, simply adding live juices (uncooked) to your water during fasting (juice fast) confers rejuvenating effects and healing of various illnesses such as some cancer, leukaemia, arthritis, high blood pressure, kidney disease, skin infections, liver disorder, alcoholism and smoking. Juice fasting literally transforms life.

HOW LONG TO FAST

The length of a juice fast can range from three to forty days. For health promotion, detoxification and rejuvenation, most authorities agree that a first-3 day monthly juice fast is all that is needed. For therapeutic (healing) fasts, however, the 4-40days range (with 20 days average) is the practice in health sanitariums in Europe. Longer juice fasts enable the body to cleanse toxins that have accumulated in body tissues from birth. More severe health conditions require fasting for 20days as it takes that long to repair damaged tissues. After four days fasting, one begins to experience enhanced energy, stamina, clear thinking and clear mindedness as well as physical healing. The appetite is suppressed by ketones until the body has finished internal cleansing. This lack of hunger may last up to 40-60days depending on whether or not one is on water or juice fast respectively.

HOW MUCH TO DRINK

During a fast, drinking300ml every 3hours is all that is needed.

WATER FASTING

While juice fasting is excellent for detoxification and health promotion because juice contains enzymes and some nutrients, water fasting is more intense and accordingly is more suitable as a therapeutic fast in conditions like cancer. During such therapeutic fasting, drinking distilled water gives best results but in its absence, spring or bottled water is the next best option. Water fasting cures drug addiction, substance abuse, alcoholism, fears, phobias, selfishness, and self-doubt (or low self-esteem).

DETOX PROCEDURES AND AIDS DURING A FAST

For the sake of completeness, the following procedures are often employed to help rid the body of toxins for health and life-long vitality

I.   Colonic irrigation
II.   Ozone Therapy
III.   Acupuncture
IV.   Massage
V.   Thermal chambers or (sauna baths)
VI.   Herbal liver-kidney cleansing formulas.
VII.   Anti-oxidants (Zinc, Vitamin A, Vitamin C, Calcium, Vitamin E, Essential Fatty Acids and Selenium).
VIII.   Multimineral and multivitamin supplements
IX.   Mixed essential oils
X.   Fibre supplements (Psyllium tablets)

FAST-BREAKING

Always break a fast with fruits and vegetables because of the high fiber content that acts like a cleansing sponge.

FASTING AND ENEMA: During a fast, natural bowel movements cease so an enema is often needed to evacuate the accumulated wastes introduced when fast exceeds 5days. Enema is done using 900ml of water mixed with drops of lemon juice. Retention time is a few minutes only, please. During fasting, if diarrhea occurs, use psyllium powder or enema to eliminate it

After concluding a fast one can replace beneficial intestinal bacteria using plain yoghurt (probiotics) which contain correct lacto-bacterial content or dates and onions.

Throughout the fasting period, plain water or mineral water can be taken when thirsty but the total intake per day (24hrs) should not exceed 1.8 litres

COMMON RULES FOR FASTING

1. No smoking or drinking alcohol.
2. Do not take even a morsel of any solid food, otherwise the gastric juice will start to work and the benefits of the fast will be lost.
3. Withdraw all drugs (except insulin for diabetes, digoxin for heart disease and cortisone for arthritis).
4. Regular work should continue.
5. Mild exercise is very helpful, particularly in fresh air.
6. Do not lie around in bed, it could be harmful.
7. Daily baths are important to wash away toxins that are eliminated through the skin.

BENEFITS OF FASTING

The human body replaces 300-800 billion cells in your body every day. And about $\frac{1}{4}$ of your body cells are in the state of disrepair and need replacement in order for the body to build new ones. It is during sleep (nightly fast) that the cleansing process is most efficient and effective. In other words, it is during sleep (or fasting) that the body under goes metamorphosis in which there is tearing down and rebuilding of damaged materials. That is why fasting is famous for its ability to rejuvenate and give the body more youthful look and attractive countenance.

In addition to physical healing, fasting enhances and sharpens the thinking faculty in the brain. Both mental and physical senses are heightened to confer emotional stability and an acute sense of well-being as well as general joie de vivre.

CHAPTER 8
RED MEAT ABSTINENCE FOR HEALTH

"Nothing will benefit human health and increase the chances for long survival of life on earth as much as evolution to a vegetarian diet"

(Albert Einstein)

Except for blood group O individuals and to some extent blood group B, the liability to fall ill at any age is increased ten-fold by consumption of red meat. The intellectual, moral and physical powers of the consumer of red meat tend to depreciate by its habitual use. Meat eating deranges the body, beclouds the intellect and blunts moral sensibilities. This may very well explain the pervading poor school performance, high rate of moral decadence as well as the high crime rate in the societies that consume a lot of red meat. For instance red meat eating is associated with high aggressiveness and violence (as seen in lions and other carnivorous animals) while vegetarianism is known to raise moral and intellectual performance in humans.

In relation to physical health, red meat consumption increases the risk of diseases like obesity, high blood pressure, cancer, heart disease, kidney disease, fibroid, cataracts and so on.

For example, when a vegetarian changes diet to red meat consumption, they tend to put on weight and their blood pressure rises sharply but when a meat eater turns to vegetarian diet he/she loses weight rapidly and their blood pressure drops dramatically.

The evil of red meat consumption comes out most graphically in the case of cancer of the colon, the third commonest cancer that affects men and women, as shown below.

Frequency of eating beef, pork and lamb	% Cancer risk outcome
< 1 per month	0
Between 1 – 2 per week	39%
" 2 – 4 per week	50%
" 5 – 6 per week	84%
Daily or more	149%

In other words, eating no red meat at all is associated with zero increase in the risk of colon cancer. On the other hand, eating red meat regularly raises the risk by a factor of about 149%. This is likely to be true of other cancers and tumors, including fibroids and leukaemia

The risk of cancerous growths in the body occasioned by red meat consumption is astronomically worsened by barbecuing, frying and grilling of red meat (suya, fried chicken, grilled or smoked fish). This is because these methods of preparing meat and fish tend to produce cancer-causing chemicals like benzpyrene and methylcholantherene which are associated with high risk of cancer and leukaemia.

Red meat consumption is also associated with higher incidence of Type 2 diabetes mellitus.

On the flipside, by limiting the amount of red meat in your diet in favour of a more vegetarian/fruitarian diet, one can dramatically reduce the risk of developing diabetes, heart disease, fibroid and cancer. For instance eating red meat twice a day increases the risk of heart disease in women. The risk is worse with highly processed meats sold in fast food joints.

Another down side of red meat eating is that farmed red meat is loaded with harmful pesticides, hormones and environmental pollutants including DDT, PCB, and so on.

In summary, red meat consumption presents the following health risks:

DISEASE CONDITION	REMARK
1. Brain Tumour	Risk increases in both consumers of red meat and their offsprings
2. Liver Cancer	Risk particularly high for roasted/grilled meat like suya and fried chicken due to harmful chemicals from the oils used to grill or fry the meats as well as the harmful chemicals from the meat itself.
3. Back pain	
4. Breast Cancer	
5. Kidney Cancer	
6. Pancreatic Cancer	
7. Colon Cancer	
8. Leukaemia	
9. Heart Disease	
10. Diverticulitis	

11.	Easy Fatiguability	
12.	Lack of stamina and endurance	
13.	Fibroids	
14.	Osteoporosis	
15.	Gout	
16.	Ovarian Cancer	Fried chicken /meat (greatest culprit)
17.	Prostate Cancer	
18.	Hypercholesterolaemia	
19.	Stroke	

HOW TO CHANGE TO VEGETARIAN DIET

Making diet change can be very difficult because of the following:

a.   Emotional association - socio-cultural

b.   Coping mechanisms – depression, loneliness, loveless relationship

c.   Physiological reason – sugar addiction

d.   Poor eating habit (late night keeping, skipping breakfast, eating fast foods)

e.   Delicious meals tempting.

It is refreshing to know that the problems with delicious meals, poor eating habits, socio-cultural and emotional obstacles can be overcome with proper nutrition education set out in this book. Once a person is fully aware of the benefits and other advantages of non-flesh diet, it takes just two or three weeks to overcome the habit of flesh-eating for instance.

Sugar addiction which is responsible for the epidemics of obesity, hypertension, diabetes and heart disease across the world takes two months or more to overcome. The obstacles of depression, loneliness and loveless marriages can be handled professionally by a therapist or psychiatrist.

CHAPTER 9
FOOD GROUPS

If one compares the human body to a car with the engine, the body and the tires as the structural components of the body as built up by proteins, then the petrol one puts inside the car to provide energy for driving could be compared to carbohydrates in human diet. The engine oil, radiator water and hydraulic fluid which are very essential for the smooth functioning of the car could be likened to fats and oils in the body. Other parts of the car that are small but play vital roles in the functioning of the car include things like fuses, bolts, plugs and nuts. These could be likened to vitamins in human diet. They are needed in very minute quantities but their absence or deficiency can spell malfunction or disease, often leading to death.

In order to appreciate the concept of eating right and applying it effectively in our lives, it is only fair to start by reminding ourselves of the functions that each food group performs in our bodies. I do not by any means want to make the reader a professional nutritionist or dietician out of this very elementary discourse. All I intend to do is to present the essential knowledge about different food groups to enable him or her make sensible and informed choice of food for health and vitality. In other words, I will try to demonstrate to the reader the different classes of food to enable him or her make rational selection of what to eat, when to eat it, and how much to eat at a time to ensure life-long vitality on a minute to minute and day to day basis.

The different foodstuffs consumed by us humans every day, fall into the following categories, according to what function they perform in the body. These include carbohydrates, fat and proteins. In addition, there are certain nutrients which are needed in very minute quantities but which are of vital importance to bodily functions. They include vitamins, minerals and fiber.

CARBOHYDRATES

Carbohydrates provide the body with the immediate energy which the body requires for minute-to-minute business of living. Carbohydrates provide the body with energy for working, walking, running and other bodily movements. The human brain also needs a steady supply of carbohydrates in the form of glucose to perform mental work. Carbohydrate, in addition has a "sparing" effect on bodily protein. In other words, as long as there is adequate supply of carbohydrate, the body utilizes whatever little protein is available for bodily repairs and growth. If, however, there is a deficiency of carbohydrate, the body breaks down bodily protein and uses it to make energy for activity. This soon leads to loss of muscle mass which manifests as emaciation. This means that eating high protein diet without adequate carbohydrate leads to ill-health. It is therefore important to eat protein along with some carbohydrate at every meal.

Carbohydrates include starchy foods like yams, bread, wheat, cassava, rice, maize, millet, guinea corn, sweet potatoes, cocoyam, Irish potatoes, plantain, and banana as well as sugary foods such as white sugar, sugarcane, and honey. Compared to other foodstuffs, carbohydrates are the cheapest foods in the market and form the staple food of most people in developing countries. Consequently, carbohydrates constitute the bulk of the foods eaten in poor societies where protein and fat are beyond the reach of most families.

Two (2) handfuls of grain carbohydrate or a portion of swallow, "the size of the person's fist coincides with the size of food that the stomach can accommodate at a sitting. Anything more than this is wasteful and even harmful on the long-term. Generally, we eat much more than we really need for health. As the Egyptian saying "we live on ¼ of whatever we eat daily and ¾ is what our doctors live on". In other words, if we eat ¼ of what we eat daily, our doctors would starve.

PROTEIN

Whereas carbohydrates provide energy for movement of the body, proteins provide the building blocks for growth in children and for repairs and replacements in adults. Proteins form the structural elements of the body such as bones, muscles, hair and nails. They also take part in the synthesis of regulatory proteins like hormones, enzymes, antibodies and haemoglobin. These are very critical for health and longevity.

Although proteins are to be found in almost all foods, they are in the highest concentration in animal foods such as beef, pork, eggs, fish and dairy products. Just as foods of plant origin are essentially carbohydrate in nature, animal foods are almost exclusively protein in composition with little or no carbohydrate. There are, however, important exceptions: some plant foods provide good source of protein and can most conveniently substitute for animal protein in food. The most important examples of plant food with good protein content include beans, groundnuts, bambara nuts and soya beans. The importance of these plant proteins lies in the fact that unlike animal proteins, they do not contain harmful saturated fat and harmful toxins. These plant proteins when taken with cereals supplement each other and become equal in nutritional value to animal proteins in terms of quality. One can afford to be more liberal with plant proteins without too much ill-effect. For good health therefore, people should derive most of their protein requirements from plant foods.

In view of the high level of saturated fat in animal protein, these foods must be eaten very sparingly (a few times a week or month). This is especially true for adults who need protein only for replacement of worn out tissues and enzymes. Moreover, whereas the human body has very high capacity for storing carbohydrates, this is not the case with proteins. Any excess protein ingested is wasted and comes out in faeces and urine except for the saturated fat and toxins. Only a small amount enters the "amino acid pool'' which is in any case an ephemeral store in the body with very little capacity for long term utilization. Products of excess protein digestion include uric acid and ammonia which are very deleterious to the kidneys and the liver; especially when excessive protein is consumed at dinner. When this continues over a long time, it can lead to kidney and liver disease. In other words, for the sake of the long term health of the major organs of your body, you should eat most protein foods at breakfast and lunch and little or none at dinner.

As hinted above, though excess proteins consumed comes out in faeces and urine the harmful saturated fat and toxins of animal proteins, however, get absorbed completely. The absorbed fat is stored in the body where it subsequently leads to obesity, heart attack and stroke on the long-term. To worsen the matter, protein from "farmed" animals – so-called agric foods – are also full of toxins like, pesticides, hormones and other chemicals that are potential contributors to cancer in the body. It is therefore important to avoid "farmed" animal protein and eat only organic animal proteins and bushmeat.

Though potentially harmful, animal proteins do provide some very important nutrients which are not readily available in foods of plant origin. These nutrients include some of the B complex group of vitamins (B_2, B_5, B_{12} and B_{15}) as well as vitamin D. It is therefore unwise to avoid animal foods altogether. A good compromise is to eat them only in a very small quantity and not frequently. For instance, liver is the richest source of vitamin B_{12}, iron as well as other important nutrients like some essential amino acids. Unfortunately, it also contains very high levels of saturated fat that is involved in premature ageing of the arteries of the heart. As a compromise, it is advisable to eat liver only once a week. At this rate one benefits from the rich store of vitamins in the liver without ingesting too much harmful saturated fat.

It is also refreshing to know that there are a few animal proteins that do not contain the harmful saturated fat and which can, therefore, be eaten more liberally without too much untoward effects. Fish is the best example of animal protein that does not contain saturated fat. The fish oil or fat is in fact beneficial to health because of its high degree of unsaturation. Regular consumption of fish and fish oil has indeed been shown to lower bad cholesterol and high blood pressure in the body. This is highly recommended for those who are predisposed to getting high blood pressure. The fish is best taken boiled in the form of pepper-soup and eaten along with the afternoon meals to help wrap up one's day.

Most chicken fat is contained in the skin, so that removal of the skin gets rid of nearly all of its saturated fat. One, therefore, could afford to be more liberal with chicken, with its skin removed. The chicken can be made even healthier by eating it either roasted or boiled as "chicken pepper-soup". Fried chicken is unhealthy because of its high oil content.

Game or bushmeat, has little or no harmful saturated fat and cholesterol so that bushmeat pepper soup is a good alternative to fish.

If for one reason or the other one cannot have access to fish, chicken or game then the best option is to get more of one's proteins from plant food such as beans, bambara nuts, soya beans, chickpeas, lentils and groundnuts. The protein from these plant foods is biologically inferior to animal protein but when they are combined with cereals like rice or seeds like sesame seeds, the resultant combination is usually as good as animal protein. Beans is especially useful in this respect. This makes the traditional Nigerian dish of "rice-and-beans" or "boiled beans garnished with black sesame seeds" an excellent combination that provide high quality protein without the hazard of saturated fat present in animal foods. Beans in combination with other plant foods, provides excellent quality protein equivalent in value to animal protein. That is why beans is often tagged the "poor man's meat".

In my considered opinion, therefore, beans should be made the staple food of anyone who wishes to enjoy a vivacious life on a daily basis. Beans can be taken in the form of moi-moi or just boiled and garnished with sesame seeds. At this juncture and with due respect, I hasten to humbly suggest that the combination of beans and sesame seeds be made a national breakfast for all Nigerians or indeed all Africans to live long healthy lives.

My suggestion is hinged on my finding that populations that have been discovered to use beans as staple food eaten at breakfast (for example British (baked beans) and a tribe in south east Africa) have been found to be very strong and sturdy people. The consumption of baked beans at breakfast might have contributed to the superior intellect and energy of these people.

There is yet another important aspect of protein that we need to be familiar with to enable us plan an adequate diet on a day to day basis. As mentioned earlier, proteins are the building blocks of the body. The individual building unit of protein is called an "amino acid". In the building process, about 20 different amino acids are utilized to form all the different structures of the body. Out of these 20 amino acids, about 8 of them cannot be readily manufactured in the human body. They have to be eaten wholesale from the animal protein in combination with plant proteins as explained earlier. These eight (8) are called essential amino acids. The essential amino acids include: valine, leucine, isoleucine, phenyl-alanine, threonine, lysine, methionine and tryptophan. But for children, it also includes arginine and histidine. Any protein food that provides all these essential amino acids in their right proportion is regarded as first class protein. Biologically, first-class proteins can support growth when fed alone to animals. Most first-class proteins are of animal origin. They include eggs, fish, meat and milk. The only plant protein that contains all essential amino acids is soya bean protein.

Proteins in which one or more essential amino acids are missing are termed second-class proteins and are referred to as being of low biological value. This is because when such proteins are fed to growing animals they do not support growth very adequately. Most plant proteins fall into this category of second-class protein. But because they often have different amino acids missing in them, they can quite easily complement or supplement each other very well when combined in a meal. This is one of the most fundamental principles of an adequate diet.

I had earlier hinted that the human body cannot store "amino acids" in any appreciable quantity for any length of time. This is in contrast to fats and oils which, if consumed in excess, get stored in the body as fat. In order to build a particular structure in the body, therefore, all the needed "amino acids" are best provided at once in a single meal, at a seating. To achieve this, one can either eat a first-class protein such as egg, milk or a combination of two or more second class proteins such as rice or beans. The process of selecting food to complement each other biologically is a very important principle of an adequate diet.

Very low protein diets cause loss of libido but first class protein restores loss of libido promptly. Proteins rich in the amino acid arginine are particularly important in this regard. Absence of arginine causes sterility in animals and low sperm count in humans. For optimum nutrition even in the so-called low protein diets, a food supply in which 10% of the energy is provided by protein is a safer target for optimum health. If the supply of dietary protein is insufficient, the cells lack amino acids for their synthetic activity. The first effect of this on the young child is slowing down of growth and eventual stoppage. Muscle wasting and anemia are prominent, although the connective tissue is well maintained. Mental disturbance may follow severe protein deficiency.

In summary, one can survive on a low protein diet for a long time (5g/day), but for overall good health, it is better to consume 10 – 15% of one's total calories per day as protein especially in childhood and pregnancy. A diet with moderate amount of protein has been shown to confer natural immunity through optimum production of anti-bodies to invading bacteria particularly in the elders. This may explain the high incidence of infection in our environment where the rate of protein consumption is very low. The important point is to consume protein of plant origin rather than animal protein. Specifically, we should reduce to a minimum the amount of red meat (mutton, beef and pork) for lifelong vitality and longevity. The safest animal proteins for lifelong vitality include the following: fish, chicken, turkey and bushmeat.

Adaptation to low Protein Diets

The tissues of the body can adapt to widely different levels of protein intake from 50g – 150g per day. This is in sharp contrast to the effect of varying intakes of energy (carbohydrate). The need for energy is fixed to the rate of energy expenditure. If the intake of energy is below or exceeds this need then inevitably the subject wastes or becomes obese as the case might be.

The ability of the body to adapt to a low protein diet is attributed to the liver. In protein deficiency the liver increases its output of protein and decreases its deamination activity for the production of urea and viz–viz. Here lies the crucial importance of health of the liver to the overall health of the person. This was graphically demonstrated in an Indian man who with chronic liver disease and also had diabetes, hypertension, premature grey hair, impotence, poor vision and so on. Soon after he had a liver transplant, his diabetes disappeared, hypertension was controlled; his grey hair turned black and vision improved dramatically.

Protein Content of Foods

S/N	FOOD	% ENERGY FROM PROTEIN IN FOOD	REMARK
1	Cassava	3.3	Poor
2	Cooked Plantain	4.0	Poor
3	Sweet Potatoes	4.4	Poor
4	Irish Potatoes	7.6	Poor
5	Rice (home pounded)	8.0	Poor
6	Maize (whole meal)	10.4	Add skimmed milk always
7	Sorghum (Guineacorn)	11.6	Good for weaning diet
8	Millet (Setanitalica)	11.6	Good
9	Millet (Pennisetum)	13.6	Good
10	Wheat	13.2	Very good except for blood group incompatibility
11	Groundnuts	18.8	May be harmful; may contain aflatoxin
12	Cow's milk	21.6	Too much saturated fat
13	Beans	25.6	Excellent
14	Beef	38.4	Too much saturated fat, hormones, pesticides and harmful chemicals
15	Cow's milk (non-fat, skimmed)	40.0	Excellent (Depending on Blood Group)
16	Soya beans	45.2	May be harmful Growth interference in children
17	Fish(Fresh)	45.6	Excellent
18	Fish (Dried)	61.6	Excellent

FATS AND OILS

While carbohydrates are the source of immediate energy supply for minute-to-minute and day-to-day energy needs of the body especially the brain, fats represent reserved fuel which can be mobilized when carbohydrate source is not adequate or is not reliably available e.g. during periods of starvation.

In addition to supplementing the energy supply of carbohydrates, fats and oils have other very important functions in the body. For instance, the fat stored under the skin serves as insulator to regulate heat loss from the human body. This is particularly desirable in temperate countries where the weather can be particularly cold. One other very important function of fat and oils is that they serve to create the feeling of satiety after a meal. Meals served without some oil usually taste dry and leave one unsatisfied. Fats achieve this function by stimulating the satiety centre in the brain. Fats also help in the absorption of vitamins A, D, E and K. They also supply the body with vitamin F or EFA (essential fatty acids), which have been proved in rats to prevent some forms of skin and heart diseases.

Despite their very important role in the body, however, fats/oils are needed in very small quantities only for the maintenance of optimum health. In fact an average person needs only 3-6 teaspoonfuls of fat per day. Moreover, most foods naturally contain oil in them, so that when one cuts down on oils one does not necessarily cut them out completely. One should therefore, try to cut down on oils and fats as much as possible. Excess fats are even more injurious to health than excess of either protein or carbohydrate. Fats should, ideally, constitute about 15 – 20% of total energy consumed in a day for optimum health.

Some authorities are towing with the idea of "no-oil" diet because of the recent findings from Harvard University and similar medical research institutes that no oil is safe on long-term use including olive oil. This new extreme view on oils will take a long time to win the taste of the average person on the street, considering the satiety, ecstatic and lubricating role of fats in our diets.

Fats and oils are classified nutritionally into saturated and unsaturated fats. Consumption of large amount of saturated fat, particularly processed fats called trans-fats is linked with disease of the heart and blood vessels (the number one killer of human beings in the world). Unsaturated fats on the other hand are less harmful. Indeed, some unsaturated oils have been shown to be health promoting when eaten in moderation. Most animal fats and oils are saturated except fish oil. Most plant or vegetable oils are unsaturated with the exception of coconut oil, palm oil and palm kernel oil. Persons who have history of heart disease or stroke in their family will do well to avoid animal fats as much as possible. This includes all sorts of meat and dairy products like cheese, milk and milk products.

Finally, a point must be stressed about palm oil. Although it is a vegetable oil, palm oil is saturated and should be eaten only sparingly. In Nigeria, this must sound almost heretical in view of the fact that palm oil is the most popular cooking oil which has been around from time immemorial. But truth must be told for those who care about their health. For coconut oil, even though it is saturated, the molecules are short and intermediate in length which renders it less harmful than other saturated fats. In fact, coconut oil is now recommended for the prevention and treatment of the ubiquitous brain disorder called Alzheimer's disease as well as prostate cancer.

In addition to causing disease of the heart and blood vessels, too much saturated fat and oils is linked with the development of certain cancers of the gastro-intestinal tract especially colon and liver.

The simplest way of avoiding too much fats/oils is to avoid eating all fried foods, and animal products no matter how daintily prepared. You must discipline yourself to gracefully but firmly say "no" to such food every time you are tempted to eat them.

Another very popular oil is Fulani butter (main shanu) which people use to improve the flavor of different dishes. It is highly saturated and should be used only sparingly. But because it is natural, it is far better than magarine and mayonnaise. Specifically, natural Fulani butter (main shanu) should be used on vegetable dishes (salads) to enhance the absorption of vitamin A, D, E and K and phytonutrients like lycopene, lutein, betacarotene and polyphenols.

In conclusion, I must warn that most unlabelled vegetable oils sold in the open markets are highly processed, adulterated, dangerous and unhealthy. It is better to insist on branded cold-compressed vegetables oils like olive oil, avocado oil, flaxseed oil, sunflower oil purchased directly from the manufacturers where possible.

CHAPTER 10
COOKING OILS FOR HEALTH

As far as nutritionists and dieticians are concerned, fats and oils in our foods are directly or indirectly associated with most diseases that affect man through the phenomenon referred to as lipotoxaemia, in which fats and oils in our diet act as toxins in the body. So that it is extremely important to know what oils and fats to eat and in what quantity; It equally important to know those oils. This can make all the   difference between a long healthy life and a short, brutal miserable one. There are fats/oils that kill, and those that heal. It is therefore, crucial to know and select wisely every time. The wise selection of oil/fats can virtually reverse most age-related degenerative diseases within two years. Especially if combined with juiced carrots and taken regular for this long.

Eating too little fats on the other hand can be unhealthy or even dangerous. Consuming less than 10% of your daily calories from fat and oils may actually increase your risk of heart disease. A deficiency fat intake can lower your intake of vital nutrients like vitamin A, D, E and K (ADEK). Too little fat in the diet

cause spiking of harmful triglycerides level in blood to predispose you to heart disease and stroke. Recent research work has shown that some important nutrients like the Vitamins ADEK and other anti-oxidants are absorbed 10 times more easily when vegetables are eaten with enough healthy fats and oils e.g. natural organic butter (Fulani), olive oil, avocado pear oil and flaxseed oil.

The total healthy fat content of one's diet should not be less than 20% and not more than 30% of the total calorie a person consumes in a day. This total fat should consist of ¾ monounsaturated fatty acids (MUFA) (olive oil, avocado oil, atili oil, flaxseed oil). Only ¼ of the fats/oils should come from saturated fats like coconut oil, and natural butter,(ghee) and red/palm oil.

Diets high in MUFA and coconut oil protect against heart disease, cancer and Alzheimer's disease. They also improve cognitive function (similar to wheat-germ and wheat-germ oil).

As a rule of thumb, therefore, the recommended daily amount of oils/fats is five (5) teaspoonfuls maximum. The different oils to consume regularly for health include: olive oil, cod liver oil, atili oil, flaxseed oil, coconut oil, natural organic butter, avocado oil and sunflower oil.

HARMFUL OILS

In the manufacture of commercial cooking oil, gasoline is first added to the oil seeds, mashed and the mixture is then heated to high temperature in order to extract the oils. This process renders the resulting oils unhealthy and often out rightly harmful because some chemicals are used or added for preservation. This is worse in the case of deodorized varieties of commercial oils where they are heated to even higher temperature leading to the formation of unnatural and extremely harmful fatty acids called trans-fats. Frying foods with these oils further turns them into deadly toxins (carcinogens). Obviously therefore, commercial oils that are commonly sold in our market and supermarkets can no longer be considered safe by any stretch of imagination.

In summary, apart from cold-compressed coconut oil, compressed pure extra-virgin olive oil, and atili oil state, avocado oil and flaxseed oil, all other cooking oils in the markets and supermarkets which have been processed in factories and do contain chemicals added are harmful on long-term use. In other words, for a long healthy life, one should stick to, cold–compressed, coconut oil, cold-compressed extra-virgin oil, locally produced avocado oil and atili oil from Jos Plateau State of Nigeria as well as flaxseed oil.

Recent research has shown that of all oils, coconut oil is the healthiest. This is based on its structural nature of having short and medium chain fatty acids. It can be heated to very high temperature levels without losing its value or becoming carcinogenic.

HEALTHY OILS

With the classification and exclusion of all processed commercial oils in the markets and supermarkets as unhealthy and even toxic, and given that palm oil, palm kernel oil and groundnut oil are not very healthful Even though they are not factory processed in some cases, we are left with the following few but very healthy oils to choose from for long healthy lives into ripe old age. These healthy oils include:

a.　　Cold-compressed extra-virgin olive oil (the darker the better).

b.　　Cold-compressed flaxseed oil.

c.　　Locally produced avocado oil.

d.　　Locally produced coconut oil.

e.　　Natural (Fulani) butter (in small quantities only).

f.　　Locally produced atili oil from the Jos Plateau

g.   Fish oil (cod liver oil)

In view of the supreme importance of the above listed oils/fats, it should be worth the while to dwell on each of them a little longer to drive the point home for their healing and protective properties for life–long vitality. For instance, these healthy oils are necessary for the body to absorb cancer fighting carotenoids in fruits and vegetables. They also improve the anti-oxidant power you get from fruits by a factor of five.

1.   OLIVE OIL (ATILI OIL)

"Olive oil is said to be a gift from the gods". The ancient Romans lit olive oil lamps before a baby is born. The lamps carried names and they named the baby after the one that burned the longest, in order to guarantee a long and healthy life. They believe olive oil has a soul of its own.

According to the Romans, "Its extreme versatility and magical Mediterranean taste transforms salads, fresh fish, poultry and vegetables into dishes that would appease the palates of the gods".

Olive oil has been crowned "King of All Oils" and some people have dubbed it "The Liquid Gold".

Today, we know that olive oil helps to lower cholesterol, lower raised blood pressure and lowers the risk of heart disease.

Olive oil is very important nutritionally because it has several healing and health promoting properties as follows:

(i)   It prevents infection by boosting immunity

(ii)   It is beneficial for liver and gallbladder diseases (including hepatitis)

(iii)   Helps in the evacuation of the intestine to prevent constipation

(iv)   It is rich in vitamin E, working to prevent stroke, improve thyroid function and increase oxygen supply to tissues of the body to boost their metabolism and health.

(v)   It facilitates the transformation of carotene to vitamin A.

(vi)   It prevents and controls cardiovascular diseases.

(vii)   It is tasty and highly digestible.

(viii)   It is very rich in phytosterols that block absorption of cholesterol present in food.

(ix)   Olive oil lowers blood pressure and blood sugar. It is therefore, highly recommended oil for diabetics and hypertensives. Men who simply replaced the domestic cooking vegetable oil in their kitchen with olive oil lowered their blood pressure by more than it 30 points in just sixty days without making any other changes in their diet. Fantastic!

Olive oil used regularly in cooking and added to salads, cut the risk of stroke in old age by about half.

(x)   Olive oil is said to prevent cancer and arthritis. When eaten regularly, 2 tablespoonfuls daily, it keeps the skin soft and velvety – so much so that one may never need to use skin moisturizers and lotions if one consumes olive oil regularly. One can use the money for cosmetics to purchase olive oil instead. The recommended dose is 2 to 4tablespoonful/day. It helps in weight loss. By way of caution: do not take more than 4 tablespoonful of olive oil per day, because of the tendency towards obesity. The best way to ensure olive oil is to add it raw to salad. One can also use olive oil on toast and   fresh bread according to blood group.

(xi)   Olive oil alkalinises the body (along with lemon juice) to prevent acid related diseases

2.   COCONUT OIL

Up until the last few years, coconut oil was grouped with saturated oils as very unhealthy and therefore unfit for regular consumption. Currently, however, coconut oil has been found to be not only harmless but to have far reaching, incredible beneficial effects for health and longevity. It is surprising that science is only now discovering the health benefits of coconut oil, even when some tropical populations that consume a lot of coconut oil are seldom overweight and have been free from modern diseases that afflict western nations. Contrary to popular belief, the saturated fats present in coconut oil are not as harmful as those in palm oil, palm kernel oil and other saturated fats. Coconut oil does not lead to increase .It actually prevents arteriosclerosis. And unlike other oils, coconut oil does not cause obesity because it contains short and medium chain fatty acids that do not accumulate in the body. Instead, coconut oil helps in the shedding off of excessive weight or morbid obesity by increasing bodily metabolism (good for obese diabetics).

Coconut oil is very useful in the management of digestive disorders including irritable bowel syndrome. It is an immune booster and has broad spectrum antimicrobial activity against viruses, bacteria, fungi and parasites. It is now used specifically to treat viral and bacterial diseases like hepatitis, herpes, SARS, UTI, pneumonia and gonorrhea. It is also useful in the treatment of candidiasis, ringworm, athlete's foot, thrush and diaper rash in babies.

When applied to open wounds, coconut oil speeds up the repair and healing of damaged diabetic foot. It is also effective in controlling blood sugar, to prevent and/or control treat Type 2 diabetes mellitus. When taken with food, coconut oil improves the absorption of important nutrients such as calcium, and magnesium. This function is particularly useful in women because they are prone to osteoporosis after middle-age.

Finally, coconut is useful in the prevention of tooth decay and gum disease.

CLINICAL INDICATIONS FOR THE USE OF COCONUT OIL

S/N		S/N	
1	Hair care – conditioner	17	HIV
2	Skin care – moisturizer	18	Oral thrush
3	Stress relief	19	Diaper rash
4	Heart diseases	20	Cancer (some)
5	High cholesterol	21	Giardia Lamblia
6	Obesity	22	Body building
7	Kidney diseases	23	Energy boosting
8	Indigestion	24	Impotence (Erectile Dysfunction)
9	Irritable Bowel Syndrome	25	Dandruff, Head lice
10	High blood pressure	26	Psoriasis
11	Immune disease	27	Eczema
12	Viral hepatitis	28	Urinary Tract Infection
13	Prostate Cancer	29	Athlete's foot
14	Diabetic Foot	30	Candidiasis
15	Dental disease	31	Infected wounds
16	Bone disease		

3.   FISH OIL

The benefits of fish oil for preventing and treating cardiovascular diseases have been well documented and studied. Eating fresh or frozen oily fish twice a week is the best way of protecting the heart.

Fish oil is also very important for brain development in the fetus, infant and child. Supplementation of infant weaning food with fish oil was found to be associated with a mean increase of 7 points on the Mental Development Index (MDI) of children.

Caveat: Fish oil in liquid form is highly recommended but fish oil capsules should be avoided.

FISH OILS WITH HIGH OMEGA -3 (HEART HEALTHY FATTY ACIDS)

(i)   Sardine (2.3g/100g)

(ii)   Salmon (2.0g/100g)

(iii)   Mackerel 1.8g/100g

4.   AVOCADO PEAR OIL

Avocado pear oil is monounsaturated and is very useful in the management of Type 2 diabetes mellitus. Adding avocado pear oil to vegetables and salad helps improve the absorption of cancer fighting carotenoidsas as follows:

a.   Lutein $\longrightarrow$ 5 x normal absorption

b. α – carotene $\longrightarrow$ 7 x normal absorption

c. β – carotene $\longrightarrow$ 15 x normal absorption

Avocado pear is a bonafide member of DABS as listed in the Appendix.

5.   SOYA BEAN OIL

Soybean oil is actually the recommended polyunsaturated (PUFA) omega-6 oil that may be consumed in small quantities (½ tsp only every night before bed) along with the listed monosaturated oils (MUFA) in order to balance the ratio of omega-3 to omega-6 (3:1) for optimum health.

According to scientific research published in the New England Journal of 1995, taking soya bean oil is associated with 9 – 13% fall in total LDL cholesterol and triglycerides.

Soya bean oil is also said to mop up pre-cancerous cells from the blood stream. And because of its high content of linoleic fatty acid, taking a little soya bean oil helps to fix memory during sleep thereby improving memory retention and recall. It is best taken 1 teaspoonful at bedtime.

HARMFUL OILS

1.   TRANS–FAT OILS – THE WORST OILS EVER

These are processed commercial oils (vegetable oil, corn oil and sunflower oil). They are often described as hydrogenated, partially hydrogenated or "deodorized". Trans-fats are even more dangerous to health than saturated fats. Trans-fats should be avoided as much as possible. They are associated with high risk of breast cancer, prostate cancer, cancer of the ovary, coronary heart disease, heart attacks and strokes.

Common food products that contain harmful trans-fats include the following:

a.	All commercial cooking oils in the market except for those listed under healthy oils
b.	Biscuits
c.	Cookies
d.	Cakes
e.	Pastries
f.	Baked foods
g.	Fried foods (potato chips and fried fish)
h.	Fast foods
i.	Candy bars
j.	All confectioneries
k.	Margarine
l.	Mayonnaise and other salad dressings
m.	Manufactured cheese (fake)-most chees in super market
n.	Ice – cream, chewing gum.

In short, almost all manufactured foods are loaded with trans-fats. Sadly, no amount of trans-fat eaten is safe no matter how small or infrequently eaten. So the best policy is to avoid all junk manufactured foods and all fast foods!!!!

CHAPTER 11
VITAMINS

Vitamins regulate vital functions such as growth, energy release from food eaten as well as the maintenance of the integrity of nerves and muscles. They are so small that they cannot be seen with naked eye. There are two groups of vitamins. The fat-soluble vitamins include vitamins A, D, E and K. These are called fat-soluble because their digestion and absorption in the human gut requires the presence of fat or oil in food(avocado or fish oil or natural organic butter). So that when a person has problem with fat absorption such as occurs in the malabsorption syndromes, they suffer also from the deficiency of the fat-soluble vitamins. Also, if one does not add natural butter or MUFA oils to fruits and vegetables at meals, he or she is not likely to benefit from these important vitamins A, D, E and K present in these foods.

The other groups of vitamins are referred to as water-soluble. They include vitamin C and the B complex group of vitamins. These vitamins do not need fat for their absorption. Moreover, being water soluble, they are not stored in the body in appreciable amounts except for vitamin B_{12} and folic acid. Any excess eaten is soon excreted from the body. And because they are not stored in the body, their food sources must be consumed daily for health and vitality if one is to prevent running deficient of them thereby leading to disease states.

Unlike the water soluble vitamins, the fat soluble vitamins A, D, E and K are easily stored in the body. So that, when they are taken in excess amounts, they can cause serious toxic side effects. The most toxic of them are vitamins A and D. They should therefore not be taken in excess amount or as supplements for a long time except for the treatment of deficiency states.

The common B complex group of vitamins include: Vitamins B_1, B_2, pantothenic acid, niacin, folic acid, vitamin B_6 and vitamin B_{12}. Each of these will be discussed in greater detail later.

The different vitamins are found in different foods. So that to get the entire gamut of vitamins for optimum health, one has to eat variety of foods every day. This is the reason why one must eat several different food items daily–the so called rainbow diet. Although almost all of these vitamins can now be manufactured from chemicals, and sold as supplement it is   still better to meet one's daily vitamin needs through eating natural unprocessed foods(except for folic acid). They are healthier and safer than proprietary vitamin formulas. However, the proprietary vitamin formulas can be of use in certain deficiency states or in situations where, for one reason or the other, a person cannot get all his vitamins from the natural sources. These reasons include among others: early childhood, pregnancy, old age, financial problems, ill-health or simply the nature of one's job. The most common reason militating against eating an adequate diet is financial problems. Most people cannot plan their finances to include vegetables and fruits. So that all persons who cannot eat an adequate diet for one reason or the other may need to supplement their daily vitamin requirements using proprietary vitamin formulas. Unfortunately, no single vitamin formula satisfies everybody's needs because the needs of different people depend on their unique dietary deficiencies. For effective supplementation therefore, one needs to study one's diet to see which vitamins are likely to be missing. This is why it is crucial for people to know which vitamins are present in which food items. For instance, if one's diet is deficient in fruits and vegetables it would be reasonable to take supplements of vitamin C and the B complex group of vitamins daily. Old people are especially prone to missing out on vitamin C and the B complex vitamins. They need to take tablets of the vitamin C and the B complex group daily for optimum health.

Finally, I cannot emphasize too strongly that it is not advisable for anyone to make it a habit of taking vitamins pills daily for health or vitality. It is wrong and may even be harmful. The best way to acquire needed vitamins is to eat a varied and adequate diet consisting of foods in their most natural, unprocessed forms.

VITAMIN A (Retinol)

This is one of the most important vitamins in the human diet because its absence or deficiency leads to serious disorders in man. Vitamin A is needed by the body for growth and maintenance of eyes, skin, as well as bones and teeth. It is also very important for the maintenance of the functional integrity of the epithelial linings of the gastrointestinal and the respiratory tract. The functional integrity of the above structures constitutes a 'barrier' to infection-the so called "natural immunity". Vitamin A is therefore essential for maintaining bodily resistance to invading organisms that could cause infection like pneumonia and septicemia, the two commonest killers of children and the elderly

Vitamin A deficiency leads to frequent infections in growing children especially respiratory, and gastro-intestinal infections. It also plays a vital role in the functioning of the human eye. So much so that its deficiency can lead to blindness, especially in growing children. Indeed, vitamin A deficiency is considered the major cause of preventable blindness in the world, particularly in developing countries. The blindness resulting from vitamin A deficiency is also called xerophthalmia. This occurs as part of the generalized keratinization of the body in response to vitamin A deficiency. The earliest symptom of vitamin A deficiency is night blindness. In the child, this manifests as the inability of the child to play in the dark. The child tends to sit still once darkness sets in. Other more florid signs of vitamin A deficiency are seen in the eyes. They include Bitot spots, dryness of the eyes,

Loss of lustre of the eye ball as well as corneal ulcers. Eventually, the eye goes blind.

Vitamin A deficiency usually develops as a result of inadequate intake but sometimes, it is a result of poor absorption and utilization in the body as a sequelto other disease conditions like measles. Children with measles must therefore be given Vitamin A treatment or prophylaxis as the case might be.

The rich sources of vitamin A, in descending order, include spinach, green leaves, zogele, yellow fruits, carrots, pawpaw, guava, sweet potatoes ,yams and liver. Others include red palm oil, fatty fish, and yellow maize.

To prevent vitamin A deficiency, one must eat one of the above rich food sources of the vitamin every day (except for liver which should be eaten once a week).

Important as it is, vitamin A is one of the most toxic of all the vitamins (the other is vitamin D). Too much of Vitamin A can cause serious disease, especially if taken as vitamin A tablets or syrups.

Fortunately, consuming large amounts of the food sources of vitamin A does not seem to cause any toxicity (except may be in the case of liver). The only problem with eating vegetables that are rich in vitamin A is the yellowish development of discoloration of the hands and feet which usually distinguishes healthy people who eat a lot of vegetables from those who don't.

Vitamin A rich foods help in wound healing as well as in the healing of pre-cancerous growths in the mouth and genitalia. Vitamin A protects against certain cancers, and also prevents childhood chest infections like pneumonia which is one of the major killer diseases of childhood. Vitamin A could also hasten recovery from measles attack.

Recent research has shown that high levels of vitamin A in the body prevents stroke and severe outcomes of strokes.

Therapeutically, vitamin A can be taken 100,000 iu per day to speed up healing of infection without ill-effects. This high dose is often effective in refractory skin diseases such as ichthyosis.

Vitamin A deficiency readily produces kidney stones in susceptible individuals. Vitamin A, apart from preventing and correcting night blindness helps the tear gland to secrete natural lotion that keeps the eyes clear and sparkling. Ideally, a person should consume at least 10,000 iu of the vitamin A daily to make the eyes healthy and bright. It prevents red eyes and eyes that feel as if they have sand inside. About 10ml of cod liver oil daily for a few weeks will suffice.

Daily requirement of vitamin A for adults is 3,000 iu per day, but for growing children and lactating mothers, it is higher (7,500 iu per day).

Children and infants cannot convert beta-carotene found in fruits and vegetables to physiological vitamin A. Therefore it is crucial and vitally important that children of this age (½ to 5 years) be given vitamin A supplements to prevent deficency that could lead to blindness and childhood pneumonia. This is especially important to start from child weaning at six months following baby friendly exclusive breastfeeding.

Cod liver oil (liquid) supplies about 4000 – 5000 i.u of vitamin A per teaspoonful. This amount is adequate for daily needs but not for treatment of established deficiency which requires high dose.(supplement).

In the prevention of vitamin A deficiency, children less than 1 year should be given 100,000 iu and those above 1 year should be given 200,000 iu once in every 6 months This has been incorporated into the National Programme of Immunization.

Sweet potatoes are a very valuable source of vitamin A in our environment. About 100g of it provides enough vitamin A for daily needs.

VITAMIN D (Cholecalciferol or Anti-rachitic)
Vitamin D is a term that refers to several active substances (vitamin D_1, D_2 and D_3) which are required for utilization of the minerals: calcium and phosphorus in the

body. Calcium and phosphorus are both essential for the growth and maintenance of bones and teeth.

Unfortunately, we have only two major natural sources of vitamin D for the human body: sunlight and liver of animals, especially fish liver oil (cod. liver oil)

The action of sunlight on the skin changes certain substances (natural sterols) in the body into vitamin D. For most people, this is the only source of vitamin D because dietary sources of the vitamin are few and not within the reach of most people. These dietary sources include milk, fish oils, beef and eggs.

In view of the fact that sunlight is abundant in the tropics, vitamin D deficiency should not be common here as in temperate countries where bright sunlight is often brief and far in-between. And it is refreshing to note that, by exposing one's naked body to bright morning sunlight for 10 to 20minutes between 7:30 and 10:30am, one gets enough supply of the body's daily need of vitamin D (200–300 iu).This can be done 2 or 3 times a week, since vitamin D is stored in the body.

Vitamin D deficiency is unfortunately very common in our society because of inadequate dietary intake and/or insufficient exposure to sunlight. The deficiency causes rickets in children and osteomalacia in adults. And because vitamin D is found naturally in very few foods, it should be added to infant formulas artificially to enrich them.

Vitamin D is the most toxic of all vitamins known so far, followed by vitamin A. In other words, if one takes vitamin D in excess amounts over any length of time he or she is liable to develop toxic symptoms which can be quite serious. As a general rule therefore, any vitamin tablet containing more than 200 iu of vitamin D is likely to cause toxicity on the long term. For instance, a level of about 200 iu can cause serious side effects in infants. Unlike in the case of vitamin A, consuming large amount of foods rich in vitamin D (fish, liver oil and livers of other animals) can also cause serious toxicity.

Vitamin D over-dose causes hypercalcaemia and kidney damage so there is no justification for routine use of preparations containing more than 200 i.u per day except for the elderly who can take up to 800 i.u. daily without any harm.

Vitamin D is lacking in commonly available food items in Nigeria. And because only a few people past adolescence spend enough time in sunshine to allow enough vitamin D to be absorbed into the body from the skin, it is best to fortify one's diet with 100 iu of the vitamin in the form of fish liver oils. e.g. cod liver oil, 1teaspoon twice a week.

Vitamin D is very essential in the prevention of breast cancer as low vitamin D levels in blood increases risk of breast cancer by 600%.Therefore to prevent cancer and many other diseases and lengthen ones life, one should take cod liver oil and liver of beef 2 times a week for life.

Optimal levels of vitamin D have the potential to drastically reduce breast cancer cases and lengthen life!

Children and adults taking cod liver oil or other vitamin D containing substances on a regular basis should have their blood checked at least once in every 3 months to rule out hypercalcaemia, a condition where the level of calcium in the blood is high and calcium gets deposited in the soft tissues of the body like the heart, kidneys and the brain. The condition usually responds to stopping the cod liver oil and putting the patient on steroids for some time.

As stated above,the daily recommended dietary allowance for vitamin D is 200 i.u per day except for the elderly who may require up to 800 i.u. daily without any ill-effect.

VITAMIN E (Anti-Sterility Vitamin)

Pure vitamin E is oil (tocopherol) which is practically insoluble in water but is soluble in fats and oils. It is found in many foods including vegetables. An average mixed diet provides about half the recommended daily allowance of the vitamin.

Vitamin E functions in the body primarily as an anti-oxidant that prevents the oxidation (rusting) of unsaturated molecules in tissues and membranes of the body. Oxidation (rusting) is a chemical reaction that is closely linked with the ageing process. This linkage has been carried to extremes by people who use vitamin E in large quantities in the hope that it will slow down their ageing process. Some commercial organizations even add vitamin E to their cosmetics in the hope that it will prevent or improve wrinkles of old age. Still others use vitamin E in excess amount to treat certain types of male infertility. All the above claims for vitamin E are at best empirical and anecdotal without scientific evidence to back them up. It is therefore unwise to take large doses of vitamin E until more information is gathered to support their efficacy and safety. For instance, in people with high blood pressure, taking as little as 400 i.u of synthetic vitamin E can cause serious rise in blood pressure. Others develop clotting disorders when taking high doses of vitamin E. It is recommended that if vitamin E is to be used at all, it should be natural vitamin E taken under medical supervision, and even then only low doses must be used: around 100-200 i.u per day. Natural vitamin E from food, lowers blood pressure as opposed to synthetic chemical vitamin E that raises blood pressure in hypertensive.

The most practical point about vitamin E is the fact that it should be consumed in adequate amounts when one eats healthy oils as recommended earlier. Fortunately, healthy oils contain adequate amount of vitamin E. The only problem is that excessive heating of vegetable oils in air as happens during frying and refinement in factories, causes serious loss of the antioxidants or vitamin E. This renders processed oils dangerously unhealthy. This is another reason why it is most unwise to eat any deep fried food the so called fast-foods.

The following are excellent natural sources of vitamin E is unprocessed wheat-germ oil and cold-pressed extra-virgin olive oil, avocado pear oil and flaxseed oil.

The recommended dietary allowance of vitamin E is 10 i.u per day for male and 8 i.u per day for female. This is easily achieved by eating one medium sized sweet potato at breakfast or lunch. Sweet potatoes is commonly available all-year round and is cheap food. Eating boiled with above listed healthy oil is good insurance against vitamin E deficiency in our families.

A recent Finnish study is reported to have shown that vitamin E and selenium supplementation improved mental alertness, sense of humour and well-being of inmates of an old people's home. It has been suggested that lack of vitamin E can speed up the onset of dementia in old people.Feeding the elderly with sweet potatoes (vitamin E) onions(selenium) and healthy oils (Atili,Olive oil,avocado pear) will prevent senile dementia.

Vitamin E is said to be useful in the treatment of Parkinson's disease, tardive dyskinesia and heart disease. It is also said to improve sexual health in men. Regular consumption of vitamin E rich foods like avocado and wheat-germ is thought to prevent certain forms of cancer.

Dr E.V Shute and his colleagues in Canada had discovered that persons suffering from some forms of heart disease made remarkable recovery when vitamin E was added to their diet. They doctors also discovered that high doses of natural of vitamin E improved or even cured Type–2diabetes mellitus. Regular consumption of the vitamin E is also effective in treatment of forgetfulness or dementia in the elderly as cited in the Finnish study mentioned earlier.

Vitamin E is an anti-oxidant which is useful in the maintenance of sexual function and cerebral activities; it also delays the ageing process in the elderly and is touted to be an anti-cancer agent.

With respect to naturopeutic practice, vitamin E is useful in log term management of chronic liver disease and diabetic retinopathy. Diabetes mellitus and heart disease .It is believed that without vitamin E,one has not started treatment of diabetes mellitus.

Although milk is a good source of the vitamin E, the best source of the vitamin E is wheat germ and wheat germ oil.

VITAMIN K (Coagulating Vitamin or Anti-Haemorrhagic Factor)

Vitamin K does not usually constitute much problem for most people because it is produced by the bacteria of the gut. It usually causes problems in newborn babies since their gut bacteria are not adequately established at birth. It is also a problem in people with liver disease who are placed on intestinal sterilizing drugs that kill bacteria. Any prolonged use of antibiotics can similarly cause vitamin K deficiency.

Vitamin K, acts by promoting the clotting of blood through its ability to increase the synthesis of prothrombin by the liver. The deficiency of vitamin K therefore causes delay in blood clotting. The symptoms include excessive bleeding and bruises under the skin called ecchymosis especially in newborns. Vitamin K deficiency manifests as heamorrhagic disease of newborn which results in prolonged bleeding following circumcision in some children. The bleeding is promptly arrested by giving the child vitamin K injection.

VITAMIN C (Ascorbic Acid or Anti-Scorbutic)

This vitamin is necessary for the health of the connective tissues of the body such as bones and cartilages. Vitamin C also functions to support the disease fighting systems of the body. It helps in the absorption of iron and the synthesis of red blood cells.It is also a powerful anti-oxidant that functions with other antioxidants to prevent ageing and age-related diseases.

The most important deficiency disease attributable to vitamin C deficiency is scurvy. The deficiency usually results from eating diets that do not include fresh fruits and vegetables on daily basis.

Vitamin C (like vitamin A) is easily destroyed by cooking and storage, therefore, foods containing this vitamin must be eaten fresh every day. Food sources of vitamin C include the following, in order of richness: Guava, red sweet pepper, pawpaw, orange, strawberries, fresh potatoes, watermelon, tomatoes, spinach, plantain and banana.

The recommended daily dietary allowance for vitamin C is 60mg per day. One can get more than this amount by either sucking one orange eating one guava fruit or just drinking half cup of fresh orange juice. It is very to meet the RDA of vitamin C in our environment.

Vitamin C has been tagged the "wonder drug" of the future because of the very wide range of its possible medical uses. Although these uses have not been unequivocally proved in every case, the claims must not be out rightly dismissed or condemned without trial.

Speculations abound suggesting that regular consumption of high doses of vitamin C can lower the incidence (75%) of certain cancers as well as increase the resistance to communicable infection. It is also touted to be of therapeutic value in some diseases such as rheumatoid arthritis and systematic lupus erythematosus. These claims have not been accepted by the general medical opinion and will remain a minority view of the profession until further controlled studies are done.

The controversy surrounding vitamin C and the common cold has been raging since the early 1970s as championed by late Professor Linus Pauling of Califonia USA (twice Nobel Laureate) who believed strongly that high doses of vitamin C daily can prevent common cold in addition to creating a general feeling of well-being that exudes vitality. The Professor used to take 2000mg of the vitamin daily until his death at 94 years old. He did it to prove that vitamin C is safe and beneficial.

I personally have found the vitamin to be very useful in aborting the common cold when taken in high doses, 400-500mg at once then 200mg every 2hrs for six doses. This works best when taken very early in the illness.

Recent work has also shown that vitamin C in high enough doses (500mg/kg) can mop up viruses in the blood; it has been touted to be of benefit in the treatment of viral hepatitis and herpes zoster. Whether or not it will help in mopping up viruses in chronic hepatitis B carrier states and HIV [+] patients remains to be proven.

Vitamin C has also been shown to improve the symptoms of peptic ulcer disease, especially if taken as vitamin C in certain foods rather than the proprietary tablets.

It also helps control the symptoms of diabetic mellitus. It is also said to restore fertility in some infertile men.

Based on a study in which vitamin C (100mg) was given to school children over a period of six months, the IQ and mental alertness of the children involved were said to have improved dramatically. This can also be attributed to its ability to improve iron absorption from food.

The common fruits that are rich in vitamin C include citrus fruits, guava, fresh sweet potatoes, pawpaw, pepper (red & green), tomatoes and pineapple. These should be consumed daily because vitamin C is not stored in the body. To worsen matters, vitamin C is easily destroyed by heat. It oxidizes easily being a powerful reducing agent. The vitamin easily dissolves into the drain when foodstuffs are washed. This means that for optimum health, the vitamin is best consumed in fresh raw foods. Therefore, taking of proprietary supplements of the vitamin daily becomes inevitable. The latter is particularly important for the elderly who should take at least 200mg of the vitamin with every meal. I personally take 400mg daily and the experience is simply exhilarating.

It is gratifying to note that the vitamin C in sweet potatoes is not destroyed by cooking, making this very ubiquitous root carbohydrate a wonderful super fool for the poor!

VITAMIN B GROUP

Vitamin B complex deficiency lies at the root of most psychosomatic illnesses such as anxiety, depression and nervous tension. A diet rich in vitamin B complex will correct most psychosomatic disorders. Such a diet should include Brewer's yeast, wheat-germ, black treacle (mazankwaila) and yogurt. Adequate Vitamin B complex is most important for outwitting chronic fatigue. The best way to do this is to consume either three tablespoonful of Brewer's yeast or wheat germ or black treacle every day,because vitamin B complex is not stored in the body.

To stay young at heart one should eat lots of foods that are rich in vitamin B complex daily, (Brown (potaoe) rice,wheatgerm, Brewer's, yeast and whole grains). In addition, one should also eat calf and lamb brains and liver once a week. Dr T.S. Gardner, in an experiment was able to increase the life-span of laboratory animals by 46.6% by simply adding the following vitamins to their diet: Riboflavin

(B$_2$), Pyridoxine (B$_6$), yeast, nucleic acid, and pantothenic acid (B$_5$). All these are present in Brewer's yeast!!! . Dr. Lerster Morrison also discovered that vitamin B complex deficiency can lead to hardening of the arteries and rise in blood pressure. Correction of the deficiency soon restores the raised blood pressure to normal, even though it took from a few months to several years for the blood pressure to return to normal. The two doctor's research outcomes underscore the vital importance of consuming vitamin B complex rich foods DAILY for vibrant health and longevity

Fresh organ tonics (liver, brain, heart and kidneys) are gradually becoming popular for general health maintenance and longevity insurance. The organs are blended fresh or half-boiled and taken with spices once a week for total health rejuvenation.

THIAMIN (VITAMIN B$_1$)

This is a very important vitamin because in its absence, the human body cannot make use of carbohydrate food eaten. It functions essentially to release energy from carbohydrate foods eaten. In addition, Vitamin B$_1$ is important for the maintenance of the functional integrity of the nerves as well as the digestive tract. The last but not the least importance of vitamin B$_1$is its appetite-stimulating action which helps us to eat well.

The richest sources of vitamin B$_1$ include Brewer's yeast, oranges, liver, beans, spinach and brown rice (ofada rice). In brown rice, vitamin B$_1$ is concentrated in the brown covering of the rice-grain. Removal of the brown-covering of rice grain in the process of milling and polishing virtually removes the entire vitamin B$_1$ present. This makes polished rice a most unhealthy choice for those who care about their health and vitality. When buying rice therefore, it is wiser to buy brown (ofada rice) rice rather than the white polished rice. Food processing in factories robs cereals of their vitamin B1 content by as much as 317%. This makes them truly poor and unsuitable for lifelong vitality. These include white bread, biscuits, cakes; meatpies etc. (the so-called junk foods).Dr. Joel Wallack in the USA strongly believes that if all humans consume adequate vitamin B1 (brown rice) heart diseases would virtually disappear.

Vitamin B$_1$ deficiency usually occurs in populations that subsist mainly on polished rice. Vitamin B$_1$ deficiency is also common in people who drink alcohol heavily. The alcohol tends to interfere with the absorption of the vitamin, leading to a deficiency state.

Thiamin or vitamin B_1 deficiency causes a disease syndrome called beri-beri. There are several varieties of beri-beri: wet beri-beri, infant beri-beri and dry beri-beri. The most dramatic effect of vitamin B_1 deficiency is seen in the heart and nervous system. In the heart, vitamin B_1 deficiency causes weakness of the muscles of the heart leading to marked dilatation of all its chambers. Eventually, this leads to heart failure. Sometimes this weakening of the heart occurs silently in otherwise healthy looking people who subsist predominantly on polished rice. This silent weakening due to vitamin B_1 deficiency, has been blamed as a cause of sudden deaths in some people who look apparently healthy on retiring to bed one evening but never wake up the next morning. This incidence is increasing with increasing economic hardship in the country. It is therefore vitally important to eat only brown-rice and avoid white polished rice as much as possible. The syndrome of postpartum cardiac failure may be related to B_1 deficiency.

The recommended daily allowance for vitamin B_1 is 1.4mg for men and 1.0mg for women.

Thiamine, like vitamin C, is easily destroyed by cooking and much of it is lost by mere washing. The habit of boiling rice and later washing it before finally cooking it again is the worst culinary practice ever. This practice must be abandoned nationally as unwise and unhealthy.

Again, like vitamin C and zinc, the human body does not store vitamin B_1 well; therefore, its food sources must be consumed daily to maintain an adequate amount of the vitamin in the body. Otherwise, a deficiency develops in a few weeks or less (forty days on average). This is one of the cardinal principles of an adequate diet that must be remembered when selecting food for daily consumption.

Any person doing very hard physical work, if placed on a diet deficient in vitamin B_1 will develop signs and symptoms of heart disease such as palpitations, chest pain and shortness of breath within four days. The human store of vitamin B_1 only lasts six weeks.

RIBOFLAVIN (VITAMIN B_2)

The actions of vitamin B_2 are similar to those of Vitamin B_1. Vitamin B_2, like vitamin B_1 is needed for the release of energy from food eaten. It also helps maintain the functional integrity of nerves. A few doctors have tagged it the "longevity" vitamin because it prolongs the life span of laboratory animals by 10%.

Apart from Brewer's yeast, vitamin B_2 is obtained almost exclusively from animal products, especially liver and milk. This makes vitamin B_2 deficiency a fairly common nutritional problem in resource-poor societies that have little access to animal protein. The signs and symptoms of vitamin B_2 deficiency include angular stomatitis, cheilosis and beefy red "non-tender" tongue, as well as frequent attacks of sore throat. Vitamin B_2 deficiency also causes scrotal and genital dermatitis, intense itching of the scrotal sac, magenta tongue, patchy glossitis and vascularisation of the tongue. Vitamin B_2 deficiency has been remotely linked to cancer of the oesophagus which is common in Africa.

Other symptoms include dry and burning eyes. Some cases of refractory sore throat respond to vitamin B_2 treatment. Regular consumption of vitamin B_2 was found to prevent cancer of the liver in rats.

The richest sources of vitamin B_2 include Brewer's yeast, liver, milk, roasted beef, chicken and eggs. Plant sources of vitamin B_2 include okra and spinach. Vitamin B_2 in milk is easily destroyed by direct sunlight. It is therefore best to store milk in containers that do not admit sunlight e.g. cardboard paper.

Unlike vitamin C and vitamin B_1, Vitamin B_2 is not affected by cooking temperature but is easily destroyed under pressure cooking.

Industrial food processing robs cereals of Vitamin B_2 by as much as 300%. This makes processed foods highly unhealthy for lifelong vitality.

The recommended daily allowance for Vitamin B_2 is 1.6mg for men and 1.2mg for women.

NIACIN (VITAMIN B_3)

This vitamin is very important for maintaining the health of the skin, lips, tongue and digestive system as well as the nervous system.

Niacin deficiency tends to occur in people whose staple food is maize and who in addition do not have much access to animal foods. Maize is deficient in tryptophan the precursor of Niacin (Nicotinic acid). Even the little nicotinic acid in maize is in a bound form therefore unavailable for absorption.

It was during the last few decades or so, that the staple food of most Northern Nigerians was changed from guinea corn to maize. This is because maize was found easier to cultivate compared to guineacorn and millet. It also took less time to grow and harvest. Unfortunately maize is deficient in niacin and this may be the cause of increased incidence of niacin deficiency disease in these communities.

The disease caused by niacin deficiency is called pellagra. This classically is characterized by four Ds: Diarrhea, Dermatitis, Dementia and Death. Before the classical picture of pellagra emerges, however, there is usually a prodrome of early symptoms such as loss of appetite, loss of weight, weakness, burning sensation in the mouth and inability to sleep well at night. The skin changes of pellagra usually affect exposed areas of the body such as the neck (Cassal's necklace), the hands and the feet.

The rich food sources of niacin include liver, Brewer's yeast, chicken, cheese, groundnut, brewer yeast, eggs, mango, brown rice, banana and guava.

The recommended daily allowance for niacin is 18mg for men and 13mg for women.

As mentioned above, deficiency of vitamin B_3causes pellagra or the pellagra-state in which the patient presents with mental dullness, dry skin, hyper-pigmentation, sensitivity to bright light, diarrhea and reduced visual acuity due to loss of central vision. On fundoscopy, there may be loss of foveal reflex as well as macular degeneration which may resemble congenital macular dystrophy. The presentation may also resemble primary hypothyroidism with low T4 but TSH is normal or low.

Vitamin B_3 deficiency also causes excessive hair loss leading to alopecia.

In children, vitamin B_3 deficiency tends to manifest as poor school performance similar to what happens with juvenile hypothyroidism. Some children with pellagra may present with frank psychosis.

In African women, vitamin B_3 deficiency may be responsible for menstrual disorders such as amenorrhoea, polymenorrhoea and menorrhagia in 80% of the cases.

When African women present with the above symptoms, it is always wise to rule out pellagra and a trial of vitamin B complex may be all that is needed to rectify the gynecological problem.

Other conditions that can be caused by vitamin B_3 deficiency include frequent or recurrent abortions and premature births. All patients with any of these symptoms must therefore be screened for vitamin B_3 deficiency.

Another curious presentation of vitamin B_3 deficiency is vulval peeling.

Vitamin B_3 is not affected by normal cooking temperature but it is destroyed by cooking under pressure (just like vitamin B_2). Readers who use pressure cookers should take note of this.

FOLIC ACID (VITAMIN M)

This vitamin is needed for the normal development of red blood cells and for the normal utilization of protein in the body. It is also used in the building of genetic material in cells.

Folic acid deficiency causes a type of anaemia called megaloblastic anaemia. Some studies have linked folic acid deficiency with high incidence of central nervous system malformation in newborns, especially spina bifida.

Folic acid, because of its very important role in blood cell development is given to sickle cell disease patients daily for the rest of their lives.

In fairly high doses, folic acid is said to effectively improve the symptoms of depression and schizophrenia when used along with vitamin B_{12}. Folic acid is also used to ameliorate the harsh side effect of methotrexate used to treat rheumatoid arthritis. It protects against cancer of the cervix. It also helps in preventing premature greying of the hair.

Folic acid is easily destroyed by cooking. Folic acid is found in abundance in fruits such as mangoes and oranges, in spinach and other green vegetables. Other rich sources of folic acid include yeast, milk and Irish potato.

 The recommended daily dietary requirement of folic acid for both sexes is 0.4mg/day.

PANTOTHENIC ACID (VITAMIN B_5 – the Confidence Vitamin)

Pantothenic acid is a morerecently discovered member of B-complex group of vitamins. Its actions are similar to those of vitamin B_6, that is, it helps the body utilize protein, fat and carbohydrate. Volunteers fed on a diet deficient in pantothenic acid soon became upset, irritable, quarrelsome, sullen, depressed, tense, dizzy and numb.

Food rich in pantothenic acid include sweet potato (richest), eggs, liver, milk and dates (dabino). Since I have already recommended that liver and milk should not be taken on a daily basis and dates are not easy to come by, the only option left is to take Brewer's yeast daily to attain the recommended dietary allowance of this health promoting and life-prolonging vitamin. This is the singularly most important reason for making Brewer's yeast the live wire of this diet. The other curious but exciting property of pantothenic acid is that it confers confidence that enables a person overcome stage fright and xenophobia particularly when taken as calcium pantothenate before the occasion.

The recommended dietary allowance of pantothenic acid for both males and females is 4-7mg per day.

PYRIDOXINE (VITAMIN B$_6$)

Vitamin B$_6$ is important because it helps the body to make use of carbohydrate, protein, and fat. It is also important in the maintenance of the health of the skin, lips, tongue, eyes, blood and nerves. It is believed that regular consumption of this vitamin will prevent and or improve rheumatoid arthritis.

Vitamin B$_6$ deficiency manifests early as "numbness" or tingling sensation in the hand and fingers. This sensation usually comes on when driving a car (for those who drive). There is also the symptom of night cramps in which the patients wake up suddenly at night with severe pains in the legs and feet. Often there's associated painful arm and shoulder. Other signs include: red, painful tongue, and excoriation of the epithelium, of the tongue: the so-called geographical tongue.

Vitamin B$_6$ has been reportedly used to treat the following diseases with some success: certain convulsive disorders in children, drug induced neuritis, hyperemesis gravidarum, drug-induced nausea and vomiting, cancer treatment, hereditary microcytic anaemia, carpal tunnel syndrome, shoulder-hand syndrome, night cramps, menopausal arthritis and premenstrual oedema.

Drugs that can cause drug-induced neuritis responsive to Vitamin B$_6$ include isoniazid, hydralazine, peniciliamine and oral contraceptive pill. Vitamin B$_6$ can worsen peptic ulcer disease so that one should be careful prescribing it for persons with history of peptic ulcer. When I tried this vitamin on myself I slept very deeply through the night but experienced symptoms of dyspepsia in the morning.

Good food sources of vitamin B$_6$ in order of richness include liver, chicken, beef, egg, Brewer's yeast, beans, tomato and fish. Unfortunately, the vitamin is biologically unavailable in cooked foods because cooking destroys it. For good daily supply of the vitamin, therefore, one should eat those uncooked foods which are rich in the vitamin. These include uncooked banana, green pepper, cabbage, carrots and groundnuts.

The recommended dietary allowance of Vitamin B$_6$ is 2.2mg for males and 2.0mg for females.

CYANOCOBALAMIN (VITAMIN B$_{12}$)

Vitamin B$_{12}$ is unique in that it contains a metal called cobalt. It is also called cyanocobalamin or extrinsic factor. Itis also unique in that it is not found in plant foods at all.

Vitamin B$_{12}$ is needed by the human body for normal development of red blood cells and for normal functioning of the nervous system. It is used in the building of genetic materials of cells in the body. This may be the anecdoted reason why some people prescribe vitamin B_{12} for the treatment of some forms of male infertility. Deficiency of vitamin B_{12} causes disease of the spinal cord called subacute combined degeneretion of the cord (SCDC), brain disease and pernicious anaemia. The nervous changes usually precede actual appearance of pernicious anaemia by several years.

The main sources of vitamin B_{12} in human diet are from animal products such as milk, eggs, and liver. Other sources include: beef, chicken, crab, cheese and honey. However, bacterial action in the human intestine produces some vitamin B_{12} which probably meets some or perhaps the body's entire requirement in normal people. Bacteria in yoghurt may be crucial here.

Fortunately, one does not have to eat these foods daily because Vitamin B_{12} can be stored in the human liver and it takes about 3 – 4 weeks to exhaust the store. Therefore, if one eats liver once a week, he will have enough vitamin B_{12} to last him for more than four weeks. This agrees with the recommendation to eat liver only once a week for health.

VITAMIN P

This vitamin was discovered by Dr. Albert Szent-gyorgyi. Foods rich in vitamin P include fresh green pepper, lemons, oranges and grapefruits.

Vitamin P is said to prevent stroke especially in the elderly, because it tends to stabilize blood vessels to prevent their disruption.

To make Vitamin P concoction one should slice two (2) unpeeled and two (2) peeled oranges and boil them together in one litre of water for ten minutes, then add 2 tablespoonfuls of honey and then boil for another five minutes. Drain the liquid and cool. Drink one glass of the liquid at every meal.

VITAMIN F (Essential Fatty Acid)

This refers to a group of three fatty acids. There is no known deficiency state in man. Normal cooking has little of no effect in the nutritional value of fats except deep hot frying.

CHAPTER 12
MINERALS

"When the diet is wrong, medicine is of no use! When the diet is correct medicine is of no need"
(Ancient Ayurvedic Proverb)

Most nutrient minerals are metal-derived elements in food which play certain key functions in body metabolism. Some are actually the same with minerals which are mined from the ground, some of which are familiar to all of us. Examples are copper, iron, zinc, potassium, vanadium, selenium calcium, manganese, sodium and phosphorus. In the human body, these metals exist in very minute elemental or molecular forms. Some of the minerals are essential for life meaning that when they are absent, deficiency diseases result. Recently it has been shown that mineral deficiencies together constitute the major cause of mobility and premative deaths in all of the world.

There are about 20 different minerals detected in the human body but so far only 17 have been found to be essential. These essential minerals include iron, chromium, calcium, potassium, manganese, phosphorus, magnesium, zinc, copper, cobalt, sodium, boron, molybdenum, chlorine, sulphur, iodine and fluorine. Although, the last four mentioned are, strictly speaking, not metals, they are also referred to as minerals because they exist in elemental forms in the human body. Furthermore, out of the 17 essential minerals, the most important as far as human nutrition and health are concerned are iron, selenium calcium and iodine because they are the most frequently missed minerals in human nutrition. Other important minerals are zinc, copper, magnesium and potassium these are the minerals most frequently involved in the disturbance of metabolism seen in clinical practice as will be demonstrated latter in the book.

IRON (Fe)

Iron is a very important mineral for two reasons. First, it is used in the formation of red blood cells, and blood is literally the substance of life. Second, iron is nutritionally important because it is easily missed in the diet and this makes iron deficiency the commonest and most important mineral deficiency disease all over the world. The reason why it is so easily missed is because although it is available in most foods eaten, its absorption in the gut is under very delicate control and regulation. Under normal circumstances, only about 10% of available iron in food is absorbed. This value increases slightly in the presence of severe deficiency or increased physiological need such as in pregnancy and growth. And because so little iron is absorbed at a time, much of it must be made available in food for any reasonable absorption to take place. For instance, although there is plenty of iron in plant foods like cereals and grains, they are biologically unavailable for absorption because they tend to form complexes with other substances present in these foods. And because animal sources of iron such as liver and meat are devoid of phytates and oxalates, their iron content is more readily available for absorption. To improve iron absorption from plant food, it is necessary to eat the food mixed in to reduce the effects of phytate and oxalates e.g. calcium rich foods help to bind phytates and oxalates to facilitate iron absorption. Iron absorption can be further be improved by eating food rich in vitamin C such as oranges, pawpaw and other fruits. Vitamin C helps to reduce iron from its ferric (highly bindable form) to a more readily absorbable ferrous state. This is one of the most important principles behind eating varied (rainbow) foods at meals especially breakfast (TABS) in order to achieve adequate diet for life-long health and vitality. For growing children, women and lactating mothers, iron demand by the body is so great that deliberate effort must be made to increase iron available for absorption through supplementation with iron tablets along with vitamin C 3 times daily. This is a very important policy issue that government needs to get involved with in order to improve the health and longevity of citizens. The diets of pregnant women and growing children should include lean or game meat in liberal quantities regularly for optimum health. This may sound contradictory to traditional belief in some African societies where children and women are given little or no meat. This culture must be condemned as ignorant and primitive.

CALCIUM (Ca)

Calcium is the most abundant mineral in the human body. In combination with phosphorus, it forms calcium phosphate which is the dense and hard material of bones and teeth.

A constant level of small amount of free calcium in the blood is essential for the maintenance of heartbeat, clotting of blood, normal muscular contractions and smooth functions of the nervous system.

The richest and most readily available animal sources of calcium are milk and other dairy products but this has recently been shown to be over-rated because the calcium in the milk and milk products is not easily absorbed compared to those from plant sources. Another animal source is small fish eaten with bones like sardine and geisha. Non-animal sources of calcium include: beans, sesame seeds, locust beans, green leaves, sugarcane, egusi, bambara nut, groundnut, mazankwaila and molasses. These are better sources of calcium for adults in view of the high salt and saturated content of milk and milk products.

Deficiency of calcium in the body can be as a result of lack of calcium or lack of vitamin D in the diet. Vitamin D is necessary for absorption and utilization of calcium by the human body. Very rarely too, calcium deficiency results from the under-activity of the parathyroid gland in the neck especially following thyroidectomy.

The most common calcium deficiency diseases are rickets (in children) and osteomalacia (in adults). These two conditions are characterized by the softening of the bones and teeth. Calcium deficiency may also impair blood clotting and cause nervous and muscular disturbance called tetany.

Recent research has shown that giving calcium tablets to pregnant women who are predisposed to pre-eclampsia can prevent the development of the disease. Some authorities strongly believe that all pregnant women should be given calcium supplements throughout pregnancy for healthy mother and child at birth. I strongly support this important modern antenatal care practice that will impact positively on the lives of future generations of Nigerians.

The calcium in our local diet is 20% - 30% absorbed. The rest (70% - 80%) is excreted in faeces. The absorption of calcium is so complex that the process is still not entirely understood. Substances that inhibit the absorption of calcium include phytic acid (in bread and cereals), saturated oils (e.g. palm oil) and oxalate (in fruits and vegetables). Too much bread consumption often leads to rickets. This is easily the most common cause of rickets seen in our urban slums in Nigeria. The rickets responds well to calcium supplementation along with cod liver oil. Children with rickets tend to have poor muscle tone and become floppy so that they are late in sitting, standing and walking. The children usually have bossing of forehead with protruding stomach similar to the appearance in sickle cell disease patients.

Calcium supplements have been found to lower raised blood pressure but only in salt-sensitive hypertensives. Calcium is also needed for muscular relaxation and regular heartbeat. Taking 2 – 4 tablets of calcium gluconate with a glass of milk at night is a better cure for insomnia than hypnotic tablets.

Up to 80% of calcium in the normal diet is not absorbed. One of most effective ways of ensuring that calcium in the diet is properly absorbed and utilized is to consume heart-healthy oils in our breakfast salad daily as prescribed in Thomas Affi's Breakfast Salad (TABS).

a)   Olive oil
b)   Cod liver oil
c)   Sesame oil or sesame seeds
d)   Flaxseed oil
e)   Atili oil
f)   Avocado oil
g)   Butter (natural Fulani)

Adding apple cider vinegar to vegetable salad as advocated in TABS effectively improves calcium absorption from food and at the same time kills over 90% of diseases that often contaminate vegetables.

IODINE (I)

Iodine is an important non-organic element in human nutrition because its deficiency readily causes disease in man.

Iodine is used by the body to manufacture a very important hormone called thyroxine. Thyroxine is made in the thyroid gland located in front of the neck. The thyroid gland is the "beauty master" of the body. Without adequate iodine in the diet, a person tends to age faster, therefore looking older than one's age. The person is soft, flabby of flesh, mentally lazy and unable to take much interest in anything and tend to lapse into "blues" often. The thyroid is truly the watchman for physical and mental health. The secretion of the thyroid gland gives the human body much of its verve and virility (so-called sex appeal). A weak and lazy thyroid gland can make sex glands lazy and an overactive thyroid over stimulates the sex glands.

The secretion, thyroxine, plays a very important role in helping the human body utilize oxygen present in the air we breathe. When a person is deficient in thyroxine, he cannot perform his usual activities well because of lack of energy. He cannot utilize oxygen to burn carbohydrate and fat so he gains weight and becomes obese. Such a person is easily fatigued (especially sexually) and is generally slow. His skin becomes dry and thick and he does not tolerate cold well because he cannot produce heat energy readily to counteract cold. He cannot think clearly and lacks the ability to concentrate and to be attentive. The thyroid gland has been aptly described as the "gland of destiny".

The activity of the thyroid gland is closely related to the activities of vitamin B_1 in the body. Dr. Russell Wilder of Mayo Foundation has found that when human volunteers do not get sufficient vitamin B_1, the thyroid gland becomes inactive. This is most graphical in pellagrins where the features of pellagra may closely simulate those of hypothyroidism. Such condition that appears like hypothyroidism but is not cannot be corrected by giving thyroid extracts but by giving vitamin B_1 along with other B complex vitamins.

Iodine deficiency usually results from lack of iodine in water of certain regions of the world. This leads to enlargement of the thyroid gland in the neck causing goiter – the so-called "endemic goiter". Endemic goiter is prevented by adding iodine to table salt in the form of iodinated salt. Another method is to give an injection of iodine in form of lipiodol 1ml every 3 years. This is one of the best methods of treating hypothyroidism to be explored nationally for the control of Iodine Deficiency Diseases (IDD).

A less common form of iodine deficiency results from eating certain vegetables that block the thyroid gland from using available iodine eg. spinach, and cabbage. It is a cause of endemic goiter found in certain regions of the world. For instance, in Nigeria, endemic goiter is common among people who consume a type of spinach that has tiny leaves. This particular type of spinach is found on the Jos, Plateau of Nigeria. It is much safer, therefore, to buy or eat spinach that has large and wide foliage.

Common foods rich in iodine include: sea foods: kelp, crayfish, herring fish, cod liver oils, kelp, duke and sardines. Other animal sources include: eggs, fortified milk and cheese. Non-animal sources include tomatoes, cucumber and spinach with large foliage.

Some other food stuffs in Nigeria have been found to cause iodine deficiency in man. These foods are said to be goitrogenic (can cause goiters). They include groundnuts, cassava, soya beans and millet. They should be avoided especially by those with blood group O.

The features of thyroid inactivity include mental dullness, dry-rough skin, high sensitivity to cold, bradycardia, low body temperature and hyper-cholesterolaemia. The symptoms are often so protean and nebulous that the patient goes from one specialist to another for years without lasting relief. The diagnosis is usually clinched when simple tests like body temperature, pulse rate and serum cholesterol total are done routinely in all patients presenting with non-specific nebulous multi-system complaints.

POTASSIUM (K)

Potassium is the "modern" mineral because in human nutrition, it has only recently been appreciated, especially with respect to its anti-hypertensive properties.

Physiologically, potassium is involved in the maintenance of electrical balance across cell membranes, which is in turn responsible for the life-force in cells. This assumes great importance in nervous tissues with regards to transmission of electrical impulses from one point in the body to another. This electrical function assumes even greater importance in the heart and muscles where electrical activity is necessary for triggering off contractions necessary for the heartbeat and other bodily movements.

On a more practical level, potassium has been found to counter-act the hypertensive effect of sodium in the body. This is a fairly recent concept with far reaching consequences for hypertensive patients and those predisposed to hypertension. Foods rich in potassium have been found to have anti-hypertensive properties and therefore should be eaten liberally by those who already have hypertension as well as those who want to prevent it. The common foods that are rich in potassium include: oranges, plantain, beans, Irish potato, meat vegetables and fruits especially avocado. I shall talk more about them later in the book.

Recent work has shown that potassium reduces the risk of stroke in hypertensive patients by as much as 40%. This is very relevant in our environment where the incidence of hypertensive stroke is high. According to recent publications, one hundred and sixty eight (168) people die as a result of stroke in Nigeria every day, while 18 stroke cases are recorded in the country every hour, and 7 people die of stroke in Nigeria every hour i.e. one person every 10minutes. A breakfast of beans, garnished with sesame seeds and eaten with vegetable salad (TABS) as I have advocated nationally will reduce the incidence of stroke and similar illnesses in the country dramatically.

A United Kingdom based cardiovascular disease expert, Tony Rudd, disclosed this at a lecture organized by Stephen James Stroke Center of Excellence in Abuja recently. The lecture was themed: "A Containable Epidemic: Developing Stroke Care in Nigeria".

Tony Rudd said that this trend would continue and even increase if urgent actions are not taken by both government and individuals.

He further said, "There are probably 160,000 cases of stroke in Nigeria every year that is 18 cases every hour. That will continue and increase as time goes by. All those people who have stroke, about 40% will die within the first month; that is twice the stroke mortality in Europe. This is about 7 people dying in Nigeria every hour as a result of stroke. This is something we must urgently do something about. And if you survive your stroke, about 60% of people will have long term significant disability. We have an epidemic of vascular disease in Nigeria. It is going to get worse if something is not done urgently about it". This is why I hasten to advocate for the adoption of a national breakfast of beans garnished with sesame seeds, eggs, fish, and vegetable salad (TABS) topped with green tea loaded with lemon peels,fresh ginger,cayenne pepper,turmeric and blackseed to prevent stroke and other cardiovascular diseases that are assuming epidemic proportions across the country. In addition we should avoid eating white rice, particularly, imported white rice. According to Dr. Joel Wallack, the incidence of cardiovascular diseases will virtually disappear if we make brown (ofada) rice a regular item on our diet nationally. If we further add Thomas Affi's Miracle Shake (TAMS) daily (See Appendix), this will promote the health of our fellow citizens dramatically and at the same time reduce health care cost in the family and the nation.

POTASSIUM CONTENT OF SOME COMMON FOODS

S/N	FOOD	mg/100g
1	Soya bean flour	1,660
2	Molasses	1,500
3	Dried fruits (e.g. Dabino)	1,290
4	Potato chips	1,020
5	Nuts (Groundnuts)	650
6	Chocolate	350
7	Fish	325
8	Poultry	313
9	Vegetables	290
10	Breakfast cereals	268
11	Fresh fruits	245
12	Syrups	225

13	Fruit Juice	178
14	Bread	168
15	Milk	160
16	Eggs	150
17	Cheese	150
18	Biscuits	140
19	Coffee	138
20	Rice	110
21	All Brand (breakfast cereal)	100

MAGNESIUM (Mg)

Magnesium has been known for a long time to be an essential element for human growth and optimum health. Person's who are deficient (90% of the world population) in magnesium tend to be nervous, irritable, quarrelsome and apathetic. As in chromium deficiency, magnesium deficiency arises from eating white sugar, polished rice and other processed foods (junk foods) from which magnesium has been removed as a result of their refining in factories. This is another reason why eating polished rice, white flour, and white sugar are seriously injurious to health. The damage done by eating such junk foods is cumulative and may take several years to manifest themselves as diseases like arthritis, heart disease, diabetes and stroke.

Magnesium is currently the most exciting of all minerals known. About 90% of all people don't get the recommended daily allowance of magnesium. The 10% of the people who actually get their daily requirements of magnesium have been found to be healthiest people around.

This is the major reason why green leaves, being one of the richest sources of magnesium in our environment, should be made a "daily-must" for a all families in the country. Examples of green leaves rich in magnesium include: spinach, ugwu, bitter leaf, moringa, baobab leaves, sesame leaves and okra leaves.

Low level of magnesium is linked to high blood pressure and atherosclerosis. Magnesium supplements have been found to be helpful in the following conditions: migraine, pre-menstrual tension, dysmenorrhoea, some cardiac arrhythmias and premature labour.

Other rich sources of magnesium include: wheat, cereals, beans, eggs, egusi soup, Irish potatoes, fruits, vegetables and dates. These are all the foods recommended in this book for life-long vitality health, particularly Thomas Affi's Breakfast Salad (TABS) and Thomas Affi's Miracle Shake (TAMS) –(See Appendix).

ZINC (Zn)

Zinc is another element, the importance of which is only recently being fully appreciated. Zinc is essential for the synthesis of protein and it enters into the action of more than 30 enzymes in the human body. It also helps the body use up lactic acid that builds up during exercise to cause tiredness.

Zinc deficiency is associated with leg ulcers, impotence (even with marginal deficiency), chronic liver disease, stunted growth in children and sexual underdevelopment. Other symptoms of zinc deficiency include hypogeusia (absence of taste sensation) of pregnancy and anosmia (poor smell sensation). Oral zinc therapy has been shown to enhance general growth of children particularly sexual development. It also helps heal ulcer of the legs by improving circulation to the legs of patients with peripheral disease such as atherosclerotic ischaemia and/or intermittent claudication. Treatment of zinc deficiency requires the use of zinc sulphate, 30mg twice a day for a week. The result is usually dramatic. Zinc is also very useful for the treatment and prevention of peptic ulcer disease. For this, zinc is given in high doses of about 200mg per day for one to two months with no serious side effects.

Zinc is present in plant foods (cereals and grains) but is biologically unavailable to the body because of the high levels of phytate in these foods. The zinc in meat and dairy products is biologically more available and is therefore the best source of getting zinc supplied to the body nutritionally. Lack of meat, eggs, fish and dairy products in the diet leads to zinc deficiency and its sequelae such as impotence. This is common in strict vegetarians as well as poor societies that cannot afford animal products. Zinc, like vitamin C and vitamin B_1, cannot be stored in the body in significant amount. For life-long health, therefore, zinc rich foods must be consumed daily.

Zinc is one of the few reasons why people must eat eggs, some meat and/or dairy products once in a while, even though such foods may be harmful in large quantities. This is especially true for growing children and pregnant mothers. No wonder then that meat-eating societies or families tend to produce taller and larger people than those that subsist on strictly vegetarian foods. For example, generations of Chinese immigrants born in America are larger and taller than their contemporaries back in poorer China. Nigerians whose diets are rich in fish (riverine areas)   or milk (nomads) tend to be less stunted compared to other Nigerians who are deficient in these zinc-rich foods (middle-beltans). Children of herdsmen, hunters and butchers are generally bigger and taller than children from other families in the same socioeconomic settings.

COPPER (Cu)

After calcium, iron and zinc, copper is the next most abundant mineral in the human body. It is essential in that it is involved in the action of many enzymes in the body including the famous cytochrome enzyme – (P-450). Copper is also essential for iron metabolism and is therefore indirectly related to blood formation. However, because it is biologically available in most food stuffs, copper deficiency is rare. Copper deficiency has rarely, been demonstrated in children with severe protein energy malnutrition who were found to have hypochromic, microcytic anaemia with leucopenia and thin bones. The anaemia and other abnormalities dramatically responded to copper therapy. Copper rich foods should therefore be included in the diet of growing children (see TAMS).

SODIUM (Na)

Sodium is needed for electrolyte balance in the body. Although sodium in the form of sodium chloride (NaCl) or table salt is the oldest seasoning material from time immemorial, several studies have shown that too much of salt can predispose certain susceptible individuals to getting essential hypertension. This is especially true for male black people who have history of hypertension in their families. Epidemiological studies have shown that human societies that consume little or no salt in their diets tend to have very low incidence of essential hypertension. Societies that consume large amount of salt in their diet tend to have high incidence of essential hypertension and their blood pressure tends to rise with age. Recent work from America has demonstrated that out of 100 people who added little or no salt to their foods, only one was discovered to have hypertension. And when people with mild to moderate hypertension leave out or cut down drastically on the amount of salt they eat in their food, their blood pressures fall significantly. In fact, some have been able to "cure" their hypertensive disease by strictly avoiding salt and salty foods (bread, biscuits, and soft drinks). In fact, the most common anti-hypertensive drugs work by removing excess salt from the body and they are called diuretics or saliuretics. They have been found to be particularly effective in black hypertensive patients.

In view of the foregoing facts, people with hypertension or those predisposed to it will do well to cut down seriously on salt intake. The best way to cut down on salt is by using little or no salt for cooking and adding no salt at all after food has been served at the table. There should be no place for the salt-bottle on the dining table of a wise family.

Another way of avoiding salt is to abstain from all foods that are high in salt including junk foods, soft drinks and bread because of the so-called "hidden salt". Other high-salt foods include milk, cheese, bacon, margarine, bread, breakfast cereals, salted groundnuts, salted popcorn, sardines, canned tomato, sausages, corned beef, meat pies, gravy-mixes, salted potato-chips, biscuits and salted butter. In short, one should avoid most manufactured products as well as all foods that are baked with baking powder. Baking powder contains high amount of salt. It is note-worthy to remember also that MSG and other similar seasoning agents have high-salt content and should be avoided as much as possible.

Sodium Content of Some Common Foods

S/N	FOOD	mg/100g
1	Bovril	5,500
2	Marmite	3,450
3	Ham	2,000
4	Corned Beef	1,505
5	Sausage	1,025
6	Cheese (Hard/Cheddar)	1,005
7	Bacon	980
8	Cornflakes	840
9	Tinned Fish	700
10	Butter (Salted)	600
11	Bread (All Types)	530
12	Salted Vegetable	415
13	Biscuits	320
14	Margarine	320
15	Cheese (Soft)	235

16	Shell Fish	180
17	Beef	70
18	Cereals (e.g. Maize)	50
19	Rice	10
20	Fruits and Vegetables	< 10

You will notice from the table above that breakfast cereals and beef are only moderately rich in sodium, with the average content of 60mg per 100g. Rice has very low sodium content of about 10mg per 100g only. This is why rice diet is highly recommended for hypertensive patients. Some authorities with extreme views believe brown rice (ofada) in particular can actually "cure" most common ailments that plague us humans.

CHROMIUM (Cr)

This is another mineral that has only recently been discovered to be very important in human nutrition. Chromium has been found to be extremely essential for glucose and cholesterol metabolism. Its deficiency is a causal factor in atherosclerosis, which is in turn the underlying disorder in coronary heart disease and strokes.

Chromium deficiency usually arises as a result of eating refined white sugar, white flour and fast-foods because the chromium in these foods are virtually removed completely in the process of their refinement in factories.

Here once again is another very concrete reason for avoiding white sugar, flour, fats and snow white rice. It has been shown that chromium deficiency may also contribute to the development of diabetes mellitus in man.

Chromium supplementation (Alphabetic) is said to prevent persons with impaired glucose tolerance from lapsing into full blown diabetes mellitus. To obtain daily requirements of chromium, one does not necessarily have to take chromium supplements but just avoid chromium depleted foods such as white sugar, and all sugar enriched processed foods (the so-called junk foods). However, chromium supplement in the form of chromium picolinate is very useful for rapid weight loss in obese per

MANGANESE (Mn)

Manganese is a very important element in fat metabolism in the human body. Unfortunately, food processing, especially in the refining of white flour and white sugar removes 40-85% of manganese in them. Animals deficient in manganese show retarded growth and abnormal bone structures. This is yet to be clearly demonstrated in man. In man, however, manganese is touted to be highly beneficial for sexual health and performance. The rich sources of manganese include: Quaker oats, millet, pineapple, brown rice.

PHOSPHORUS (P)

About 70% of phosphorus is found in bones combined with calcium as calcium phosphate and 30% is in the tissue.

It is involved in the storage of energy rich compounds like ATP (Adenosine Triphosphate) and ADP (Adenosine Diphosphate) inside cells.

It is an important cellular component of RNA and DNA. Most of the B group of vitamins only perform their co-enzymic functions when combined with phosphorus in the form of phosphates.

High protein foods such as meat, poultry, fish, egg, milk and cheese are rich sources of phosphorus; green vegetables such as spinach, cabbage and lettuce are moderate sources. Some foods that are rich in phosphorus have been said to be great aphrodisiacs. These include sea foods, termites, beans, beniseeds, red guineacorn, dates, baobab leaves, and sesame leaves.

FLUORIDE (F)

Fluoride is an essential inorganic element in human nutrition. Fluoride is important in helping the body to build healthy teeth that are resistant to decay or dental caries.

Minute traces of fluoride are found in all foods, but the quantity is too small to meet the requirements of preventing tooth decay. On the other hand, water that contains too much fluoride causes permanent mottling of teeth. The optimum water concentration of fluoride necessary for good teeth is one part per million.

Fluoride is often added to drinking water at a concentration of one part per million (1ppm) to prevent dental caries. The process of adding fluoride to water is called "fluoridation".

Unfortunately, recent evidence suggests that fluoridation of water has little direct effect in reducing tooth decay in adults. But children raised on fluoridated water develop resistance to tooth decay which carries over into adult life.

Where fluoridation of water is not possible, or is not available, dentists may apply fluoride solutions directly to a child's teeth beginning as soon as the first teeth appear, and repeat this every 3-4 years until the child is 13 years old. This has been found to reduce dental caries dramatically in children. (See your dentist for further guidance and application).

Tooth pastes containing fluoride may prove effective as well, but the dentist should be consulted before any fluoride toothpaste is used, since any slight excess fluoride can cause mottling of teeth (dental fluorosis). Moreover, like most medicines, fluoride in large amount is a poison. This is one more strong reason why one must not brush his teeth with fluoride tooth paste.Moreover because flourida has been shown to be one of the most potent immune destroyers in our environment,flourida tooth pastes should be divided altogether especially that fluoride tooth pastes do not prevent dental caries in adults. A surer way of keeping the teeth clean and bright is to use the local chewing stick prior to brushing with herbal proprietary toothpaste every time. This may be repeated two or three times a day for best results and particularly as the last prep before retiring at night.

CHAPTER 13

FIBRE

"Fibre, fibre, burning bright..."

(Anonymous)

Fibre or roughage refers to the woody part of plant food which human beings cannot digest and absorb but which has recently been reappraised as being of fundamental importance to health and vitality. It is the structural constituent of the cell wall that makes up the supporting structure of plants. Human beings and carnivores do not have the enzyme that enables cattle and sheep digest cellulose. Man can therefore only utilize cellulose indirectly through eating the meat of animals like as cows and sheep.

The undigested plant material or fibre constitutes the bulk of the faeces excreted daily. There has been a recent upsurge in scientific interest in fibre as a result of the discovery that it plays a vital role in health and vitality. The fundamental value of fibre is attributed to the fact that it helps exercise and tone up the muscles of the bowel. It was Herodicus of Selymbria who observed long ago "that a man, whose bowels move regularly and normally, will live very long". And I wish to add that based on available epidemiological records, such a person is likely to live a life that is vivacious and sparkling from day to day. The person's life remains unpunctuated by those irritating illnesses that characterize the lives of those who eat little or no fibre. Fibre tends to reduce intestinal transit time thus preventing long stasis of faeces in the body. Long stasis of faeces in the colon and rectum has been associated with the formation of certain harmful substances or toxins that are carcinogenic, and can cause cancer of the colon and rectum. This hypothesis or theory is supported by epidemiological records which have shown that the incidence of cancer of the colon and rectum is highest in populations that eat highly refined white sugar as well as highly processed low fibre foods – so-called junk foods – found in fast food joints and eateries.

Generally, African diets contain high amount of fibre that makes their stools bulky compared to stools of people who eat little fibre. This leads to lower incidence of diseases like cancer of the colon and rectum, appendicitis, diabetes mellitus, gallbladder disease, haemorrhoids and varicose veins. High fibre diet also protects against obesity because it reduces the absorption of excess fat from food eaten. I have personally observed that high fibre foods help control peptic ulcer disease by producing long remission and possible cure.

The richest sources of fibre include green peas, dried fruits,(dates) whole grain cereals, brown rice, guineacorn, millet, nuts, fresh fruits, beans, brown rice and vegetables. The daily requirement for fibre of 30g/day can be met by eating any of the following in one day:

1.   One serving of whole grain cereal. (E.g. plate of rice and beans).
2.   Two servings of vegetables (e.g. vegetable salad).
3.   Two servings of fruits. (Two oranges or one medium pawpaw or 3-4 guavas).
4.   Sweet potato (medium)

The only root crop which is rich in fibre is sweet potato. This makes it a most complete food indeed and must be made the cornerstone of our super-nutrition diet in the country. Farmers should be encouraged to grow sweet potatoes on commercial basis and Nigerians be educated to eat them daily preferably garnished with sesame seeds (black, white or yellow)

Examples of fibre rich foods include:

I.   Apples: take one before breakfast and one before bed-red apples best (wash very well with soap or apple cider vinegar before consumption)
II.   Orange (remember blood group)
III.   Quacker oats
IV.   Beans
V.   Green peas: the richest in fibre

Examples of fibre supplements include:

I.   Psyllium 2 sp daily
II.   Curamin 2000
III.   Flaxseeds 1-2 sp daily

There is no exact Recommended Daily Allowance for dietary fibre, but most authorities recommend an average of 20 – 35g per day.

It is best to get your fibre from daily food but if you have medical problems like or high risk of heart disease, you may need to take fibre supplements such as psyllium (metamucil).

Good Sources of Dietary Fibre

S/N	Food Item	Serving	Calories	Fibre Content (g)
1.	Oatmeal	1 cup	108	3
2.	Brown Rice	1 cup	230	5
3.	Baked Beans	½ cup (cooked)	155	9
4.	Lima Beans	½ cup (cooked)	64	5
5.	Spinach	3½ oz	22	3
6.	Carrot	1 medium	30	4
7.	Tomato	1 medium	20	2
8.	Green Pepper	½ cup	10	1
9.	Sweet Potato	1 medium	160	3
10.	Apple (with skin)	1 medium	81	4
11.	Banana	1 medium (x2)	230	3 x 2
12.	Almond	10	79	1
Total			1125	46

CHAPTER 14
SUPPLEMENTS AND HEALTH

"When it comes to eating right and exercising, there's no 'I will start tomorrow' for tomorrow is a disease"

(Terri Guillemets)

Do I need to take food supplements?

The answer is a capital YES! You can't afford not take them! In fact, the most intelligent decision a person can ever make is to take vitamins and mineral supplements daily. They are the best anti-aging insurance policy one can ever take.The next pertinent question is in what form should we take the supplement? The answer is avoid chemical "supplements and stick to natural nutrient-dense superfoods or herbal supplements.

Also, are supplements safe? Again, the answer is another capital, YES! They are safe and quite harmless as long as they are non-chemical,proprietary natural nutrient-dense superfoods or herbal supplements.As the name implies, supplements are supposed to be "added to" an adequate diet not to replace a faulty diet. The first thing to do therefore is to get your diet correct as in the following ways:

➢ Eat according to blood group

➢ Eat 80% of your food raw

➢ Eat healthy oils

➢ Eat some tree nuts/seeds daily

➢ Eat high quality protein daily (10% of total energy requirement for the day)

➢ Eat complex starch carbohydrate daily (70% total energy requirement)

➢ Eat sparingly $\frac{1}{4}$ of what you eat now (calorie restricted)

➢ Take Thomas Affi's Miracle Shake (TAMS) at lunch regularly

➢ Avoid deep-fried foods

➢ Avoid fast foods

➢ Avoid soft drinks

➢ Avoid junk foods

➢ Avoid alcohol, coffee and tobacco

If after you have done all the above, and still you feel you still need supplements, proceed as follows:

1. Start with foods rich in vitamins and minerals

2. Add protein meal replacements

3. Add healthy oils/fatty acids

100

4. Add Probiotics/Prebiotics
5. Creatine for those who desire body building
6. Amino Acids – arginine, leucine, glutamine (e.g. seafoods,sea salt ,Brewers' yeast(yeast powder),liver,cod-liveroil), histidine.
7. Lecithin granules (the supplement from soya products) – excellent for brain health
8. Honey and Honey productions (Royal jelly,Bee vollen)
9. Spices-Tumeric,milk thistle,cinnamon,thyme,tamarind,cayenne pepper,ginger.

SOME RECOMMENDED FOOD SUPPLEMENTS

S/N	Name
1	Bee Pollen
2	Male Virility Complex
3	Male Ultimate Adams Desire
4	Milk Thistle std Ext
5	Cayenne Pepper std Ext
6	Grape Seed Std Ext
7	Green tea Std. Ext
8	Co - Q10
10	Forever Bee Pollen
11	Forever Bright Tooth gel
12	Memory Enhance Tabs
13	Eyebright
14	40+ for Men
15	Rev-up Capsules (Horny Goat weed)
16	Cal-C-Mag
17	Double Power
18	Zinc Tablets
19	Pomegranate-Extract
20	African potato
21	Immune Booster
22	Defender capsules
23	Zinc Supplements
23	Chitosan for DM/back ache/obesity
25	Vigour - Rouser

| 26 | Cordyceps |
| 27 | Vitality Softgel |

ROYAL JELLY: take 1 pack of 30 a month, then rest for 2 months

1. Restores failing eye sight
2. Makes hands stop trembling
3. Preserves the beauty and charm of women till ripe old age
4. Makes bones stop aching at menopause
5. Treats sterility, impotence and frigidity in women
6. Turns white/grey hair to black (take along with Brewer's yeast + liver and PABA)

CHAPTER 15
FOODS AND THEIR VALUES

(Hausa Proverb)

In this chapter, I shall go on to elucidate the type and proportions of nutrients present in each food .The so-called"food values". This knowledge is very necessary if we are to make sensible choice of what we should eat, when we are to eat them and how best we should eat them in order to ensure that they may confer on us the highest level of health and vitality we all aspire to on a day to day basis.

It is a great privilege indeed that one knows the nutritional value of each food item one puts into one's mouth at every meal, every day of the week and all year round. This intellectual achievement in a way deifies us and sets us miles apart from those who are ignorant and/or do not care. The difference is physically, mentally and psychologically all very clear.

In view of the extreme importance of the topic, therefore, I have taken time to spell out the nutritional values of each food item alphabetically for ease of reference only.

ACHA

Acha is a grass cereal grown mainly in the middle belt region of Nigeria. It is used as a popular food by the people native to these areas.

Functionally, acha is a carbohydrate with little protein and fat. The protein in acha is slightly inferior to that of other cereals such as maize, guineacorn, rice and millet. Acha is particularly poor in minerals. In view of its poor nutritional profile therefore it is unwise to make acha a staple food as is advocated by some health workers as being the best carbohydrate of choice for diabetics. It may be alright if it is eaten once in a while for the sake of variety only. The old teaching that diabetics should make acha their mainstay food is highly erroneous and partly explains why some diabetics on this restrictive diet had done poorly and died prematurely.

APPLES

The old adage which says that "an apple a day keeps the doctor away", is not just old time folklore but is a veritable truism that has since been confirmed by science. An apple is a low caloric food (80cal/apple) which is very rich in potassium (the anti-hypertensive mineral) and also a wonderful source of fibre. The fibre in an apple is largely pectin,Eating red apples ($\frac{1}{2}$) in the evening is said to remove harmful heavy metals from the body.

Recently, it has been discovered that apples grow very well on the Jos Plateau. Apple is an excellent food for weight loss, especially for those who want to lose weight or those who want to maintain their present weight. Apple is also rich in phytogen and quercetin that is said to extend life expectancy.

BAMBARA NUTS (GURJIYA)

The protein of bambara nuts is of high biological value with high levels of the amino acid lysine, cystine and fair amounts of sulphur containing amino acids such as methionine. It is also rich in the minerals – calcium and iron, though it is poor in phosphorus and is low in fibre.

In view of its outstanding nutritional profile, bambara nut mixes well with other cereals like guineacorn, millet and rice in order to achieve an adequate diet. Methionine and cystine are known to have protective effects on the liver and they are particularly recommended for senior citizens.

From personal experience, eating bambara nuts regularly improved my vision and general well-being. I personally recommend it for regular consumption for life–long health and vitality into ripe old age. It can be taken as okpa wrapped in leaves (not in polythene bags). It can also be boiled and garnished with black or brown sesame seeds to replace black-eyed pea in TABS.

BANANA

Banana is a fruit that is rich in potassium and vitamin B_6. It is also fairly rich in magnesium and vitamins A and C. Given its good nutritional profile, banana is a good food for children. However, because of its high calorie content (115cal/banana) it should be eaten sparingly by those watching their weight. It should also be avoided by persons with kidney failure, because of its high potassium content. Banana is a great antihypertensive in view of its very high potassium content.

Because cooking destroys vitamin B_6 so that banana is about the best source of this vitamin in our environment because it is eaten raw.

Banana also contains a good amount of the mood elevating amino acid– tryptophan which when taken at breakfast helps to brighten one's day. I personally take two banana fingers with boiled beans garnished with black sesame seeds daily as breakfast. It is based on my wonderful experience with this combination that has compelled me to suggest that it be adopted nationally for the benefit of all of my compatriots.

BAOBAB LEAVES

Baobab leaf also called miyan kuka in Hausa is very rich in fibre, calcium, iron and phosphorus. It isan excellent food for growing children, pregnant women and lactating mothers.The calcium content is one of the highest of all local foods in the country.

BEANS (Cowpeas/Black–eyed peas)

This is a most wonderful superfood also called (magic bullet) that must be made the mainstay food in our super-nutrition programme nationally. It is a most complete and balanced food. It is rich in protein, healthy fat, complex carbohydrate, minerals, vitamins, fibre and lecithin.

The protein in beans is of very high biological value. So much so that it is accepted nutritionally as a good substitute for animal protein. The nutritive value of beans closely resembles those of whole grain cereals but there are important differences which makes beans a most valuable food to complement cereals, especially rice. Beans has higher protein content than cereals (28/100g dry wt). The biological value of beans protein is not first class, owing to their low content of sulphur-containing amino acid – methionine, hence the need to combine it with eggs at each meal (TABS). On the other hand, beans is rich in lysine of which many cereals (including brown rice) are deficient. So that a combination of beans and cereals produce protein of very high quality equivalent to that of animal protein. When combined with cereals like brown rice, the resultant protein is first class. This makes the traditional Nigerian dish of rice and beans an excellent meal for breakfast and lunch!

Beans is rich in potassium and moderate in sodium. This makes beans the perfect food for the hypertensive, the diabetic and those with heart disease. It is also good for those who want to prevent hypertension.

Beans contain some soluble digestible carbohydrate but it is low in fat. The fat in beans is polyunsaturated healthy fat. Beans is a perfect food for people with weight problem. The calorie content is 110cal/cup making it a high calorie food. Beans has a fair amount of vitamins A and B though deficient in riboflavin (B_2). It is also deficient in vitamin C, so it must be accompanied by foods that contain large amount of vitamin C such as red sweet pepper, guava, pawpaw, carrots, mangoes (DABS). If fruits are hard to come by, 2 tablets of proprietary vitamin C with each meal would be most expedient. Proprietary vitamin C is indicated at a dose of 200 to 500 mg 3 times a day for lifelong health and vitality. NUTRI–C for children for example is great nutritionally as a good source of this most important anti-oxidant that helps in the absorption of iron in children's food.

In view of the beautiful nutrient profile of beans, it is highly recommended to be made the backbone of the life-long vitality diet advocated in this book except for persons with blood group B, who may take lima beans and bambara nuts instead. It can be taken morning and afternoon. It can be eaten boiled or made into beans porridge or beans soup.

Finally, beans is rich in soluble fibre that helps lower raised levels of blood glucose! Recent scientific research has confirmed that the fibre of beans which is soluble significantly lowers blood glucose level in diabetics. Beans is truly an all-round food item that is highly recommended for daily consumption at breakfast – one of the so-called "daily-musts" for life-long health and vitality.

In fact a group of Tibetan natives who subsist virtually on beans alone have been found to live to 150 years on average in perfect health. This is a great lesson indeed for Nigerians and all persons wishing for life-long health and vitality into ripe old age.

In addition to the nutritive value of beans, it has been shown to help maintain or even improve sexual potency in men, because it promotes erection. According to the Latin poet, Martial (AD 104) "if your wife is old and your members languid beans can do more than fill your belly". And from western Georgia in Russia, a man aged 128 years old once said, "If you want to improve your health quickly, eat beans".

The major precaution with beans is that if one is to eat beans daily as recommended, it is advisable to soak the beans overnight to remove the natural toxins present in the beans such as anti-haemagglutinins and cyanogens. To further reduce the levels of these harmful natural toxins in bean meals, the water used for boiling the beans should be thrown away after the beans is "done". This may entail the loss of some vitamins, but it is preferable to consuming high concentration of these natural toxins regularly.

[NOTE: This soaking, boiling and throwing away of water should never be applied to brown rice because the vitamin loss is unacceptably too serious and in any case rice does not contain serious natural toxins like beans].

BEEF (LEAN)

Lean beef is first and foremost a good source of protein. It is also an excellent source of iron. It is rich in vitamin B_{12}, biotin, and zinc. Beef has the lowest sodium content of all meats. But unfortunately, beef also has the unhealthiest fat and if farmed,is loaded with potential harmful hormones, pesticides, herbicides and antibiotics.So if you beef stick to that of free-range grass-fed and organic beef.

In view of its rich protein and iron content, beef in moderation is highly desirable for growing children, pregnant women and lactating mothers. However, because of its high saturated fat content ,it should be eaten only sparingly by adults (about 0.5g/kg/day). This is equivalent to the size of a typical piece of meat served with a plate of rice and beans in a "buka" by "mama put" Any orders for extra-meat or pepper soup is not only wasteful but is highly injurious to one's health and vitality.

Beef is also a very high calorie food (222cal/28g) making it most unsuitable for people with weight problem and all those who care for maintaining ideal body weight.

Lean beef (grass-fed) is particularly good for persons with blood group 'O' but it should be avoided by persons with other blood groups.

BEETROOT

It is the secret weapon of sports stars and it can help stave off cancer. Its secret is in its high content of nitrates. It contains 20times the nitrates of other vegetables.

Nitrates in beetroot lower blood pressure. Drinking just 250ml of beetroot juice a day dramatically lowered blood pressure for 3 hours and 500ml of beetroot juice dropped blood pressure for 6 hours. The higher the blood pressure the greater the drop.

Nitrates in beetroot are converted to nitric oxide which relaxes and widens the blood vessels allowing blood to circulate freely to lower raised blood pressure.

Nitrates in beetroots also increase stamina, prevent fatigue and improve sex performance every time; it also boosts endurance as well.

Beetroot boosts brain performance due to increased blood flow to the brain vessels and prevents dementia and Alzheimer's diseases. The red pigment in beetroot (betacyanin) is a powerful anti-oxidant that fights cancer in the body, especially prostate and breast cancer.

Beetroot is very high in fibre that helps to regulate blood sugar and fight diabetes and cancer. To be hale and hearty always, therefore, one is strongly advised to take beetroot and beet leaves daily. The above mentioned wonderful benefits informed the special place accorded beetroot occupies in the TABS.

CABBAGE

Cabbage is highly recommended and should be eaten regularly (TABS) for the following reasons:

First and foremost, it is a good source of fibre. Second, cabbage is a rich source of vitamins A and C as well as folic acid and coenzyme Q10.

Regular consumption of cabbage has been linked with reduced risk of certain cancers. It is cheap and available almost all year round in this country.

Cabbage is a low calorie diet (30cal/cup) making it an excellent filler food for slimmers and those who want to prevent obesity.

In view of the unhygienic method of growing and harvesting cabbage like most other vegetables in the country, I strongly advise that it should be thoroughly washed preferably with apple cider vinegar before eating. It should be boiled a little or steamed before eating. Eating raw vegetables in salads is about one of the easiest ways of contracting typhoid fever due to heavy contamination during their harvesting.

A little caveat, however, is the fact that raw cabbage contains a significant amount of goitrogenic substances that preclude its consumption on a daily basis. However, boiling removes most of these harmful substances present in cabbage, rendering it safe for consumption on a regular basis.

CARROTS

Carrot is another wonderful food that is highly recommended in the life-long vitality diet for the following reasons.

First, carrot is a low calorie food (50cal/cup) making it an excellent filler food for weight-watchers and those who care about their health.

It is a great source of two very important nutrients: potassium and vitamin A. Consumption of carrots is associated with reduced incidence of chest infection in children because of its high vitamin A levels. It should be blended and given to children at breakfast regularly along with other vegetables (TABS).

Regular consumption of carrot, like other fresh vegetables is linked with reduced incidence of certain cancers of the gastrointestinal tract and skin.

The high potassium content of carrot makes it an invaluable food item for persons with high blood pressure and those who want to prevent it. Carrots are fairly cheap and available almost all year round.

Boiling of carrot is necessary before consumption for two reasons: it helps prevent transmission of diseases since they are unhygienically harvested; and the vitamin A in carrot is more readily available for absorption when carrot is boiled before eating. Boiling or cooking also disrupts the walls of the fibre in carrots thus making it more easily digestible.

Eating carrots regularly will make a person's palms and soles turn slightly yellowish but this is a hallmark of good health and vitality which distinguishes the healthy vegetarian from the rest of the people. If possible, carrots should be consumed daily as part of the life-long health and vitality program. It is often referred to as the "miracle vegetable" in view of its remarkable healing properties. Some naturopeutic doctors assert that regular consumption of carrot juice can prevent, control or even cure most degenerative diseases in one year if it is taken consistently.

CASHEWNUT

Cashew nut is a good source of iron, vitamin A, folic acid, protein and copper. It is also rich in phosphorus. It is therefore, a very good food for "snacking". So, instead of taking meat pie or cakes or even roasted groundnuts for snacks, it is much better to buy cashew nuts for health and vitality. It is rich in zinc, manganese, copper and arginine, therefore, excellent for sexual health.

CASSAVA

Cassava is almost pure carbohydrate with only 1% protein and no fat at all. Cassava when poorly prepared, releases cyanide which can kill instantly (if in high enough concentration). Even at less toxic levels, cyanide in cassava can poison the body slowly over many years and lead to certain diseases such as tropical ataxic neuropathy, diabetes and peptic ulcer, first described by Professor Osuntokun at the University of Ibadan as being prevalent amongst chronic cassava eaters. Recently, reports from India confirm that the problem of peptic ulcer disease is confined to the southern states where cassava is their staple food.

Recent work from Ibadan has shown that cassava consumption in any form is the commonest cause of exacerbation of peptic ulcer disease in Nigeria, so that any person with ulcer should avoid cassava and cassava products for long term-remission.

Prof. Nwokolo at Enugu had linked chronic cassava consumption to topical pancreatitis syndrome which is a form of diabetes mellitus. In addition, cassava has been shown to be goitrogenic, particularly in people with blood group O.

All the above points go to show that cassava and its products are unwholesome food items and should be avoided by all who care about their health. The Obasanjo national policy of insisting on cassava bread was uninformed and ill-advised (nutritionally speaking) in view of the potential toxicity of cassava and its products.

CAULIFLOWER

Cauliflower is a good vegetable to eat on a regular basis for two major reasons. First, it is a very low-calorie food (30cal/cup) that is good for weight watchers.

Secondly, regular consumption of cauliflower, like most vegetables is associated with reduced risk of some cancers. Moreover, it is rich in vitamin C, folic acid and biotin. Regular consumption of cauliflower is said to boost intellectual performance as claimed by the American renowned writer Mark Twain who had attributed his prodigious creativity to the regular consumption of cauliflower.

CHEESE

This is a product of milk which is a very good source of protein and calcium. It is also a rich source of potassium, zinc and vitamins A, B_{12} and niacin.

Cheese, like other milk products, is very good for pregnant women, lactating mothers and growing children. But because of its sodium content, it is highly undesirable for non-pregnant adult nourishment. In fact, persons suffering from hypertension and those on salt restricted diets are well-advised to avoid milk and milk products,including cheese.

For child nutrition, however, cheese is great. It can be sliced or grated and added to a young child's food in the form of sandwich or just sprinkled on food such as rice and beans.

When buying cheese it is advisable to select hard or semi hard cheese; and the colour should be rich yellow. It is hygienic to remove all moulds before use. Soft cheese is likely to be fake cheese made from trans-fat margarine as is sold in supermarkets across the country. They are literally well-packaged poisons which must be avoided as much as possible.

CHICKEN

Chicken is an excellent protein source for both children and adults in view of its low fat content. The fat of chicken is concentrated mainly in the skin, so that removal of the skin before cooking gets rid of most of its saturated fat.However, some agricultural chickens retain much of their fat even after the skin has been removed. Fortunately, the fat in chicken is monounsaturated, thereby causing little change in plasma cholesterol. Moreover, chicken is rich in carnosine, a substance now promoted as being very good for health and longevity.

When buying chicken, it is better to buy plucked or dressed chicken than live birds because ¼ to ⅓ of the weight of a live bird is contributed by its feathers and intestines.

More recent studies have shown that regular consumption of chicken bones drastically reduces the incidence of acute exacerbations of rheumathoid arthritis.

COCOA AND ITS PRODUCTS

Cocoa is produced mainly in the western part of Nigeria. It is used to produce chocolate and some non-alcoholic beverages.

These food items are high in calorie in addition to being high in fat. The combination of high fat and high calorie content of cocoa products make them ideal drinks in cold temperate countries where people drink them to keep warm. In hot tropical countries like Nigeria, however cocoa products are most undesirable because they are highly fattening and readily cause obesity in susceptible individuals. They should be avoided as much as possible, especially, by pregnant women to prevent large babies that often lead to difficult labours and subsequent high rates of Caesarean sections, particularly, in primigravidae.

Cocoa products also contain an alkaloid called theobromine, which is very similar to caffeine in tea and coffee. Theobromine, like caffeine, is a central nervous system stimulant. For this one more reason, cocoa products should be avoided if possible because their regular consumption is unhealthy. The methylxanthines (caffeine and theobromine) destroy vitamin C in the human body and interfere in the growth of children, and is very unhealthy for pregnant women and their unborn babies.

COCONUT OIL

Coconut oil, like palm oil, is highly saturated. However, it is better than palm oil because its molecules are made of short and medium chains that are make it harmless compared to other saturated fats. Moreover, recent work has shown that coconut oil prevents and treats Alzheimer's disease if consumed in small amounts regularly.Its also good for weight loss in obese persons.

COCOYAM (TARO)

Cocoyam is a very good food indeed (except for blood group O persons). Although classified as carbohydrate, it is rich in protein and minerals. Cocoyam is a wonderful food for growing children because its minerals are much more available biologically compared to those of cereals.

For instance, the iron content of cocoyam is 93% available for absorption compared to 30% availability from cereals like guineacorn, wheat and acha. Its calcium content is 90% available, compared to 30% availability of calcium in cereals like, maize and guineacorn. Cocoyam should be served with plenty of fruits and vegetables to make for an adequate diet in terms of vitamins and fibre.

COTTON SEED OIL

The oil from cotton seed is poly-unsaturated and therefore good for health. It is also rich in vitamin E. It is fairly rich in minerals as well. Unfortunately, if it is not properly prepared, it may contain toxic impurities that may prove harmful in the long term.

DATES (DABINO)

This fruit is low in calorie (22cal/dates), and rich in potassium, magnesium and niacin. It is also a good source of iron. In view of its beautiful nutrient profile, dates should be eaten regularly for health and vitality. A little of it goes a long way. It is also a high phosphoric item that helps improve sexual desire and performance. Taking five dates soaked overnight in goat milk (or any milk) or plain water taken in the morning and repeated in the evening for 30 days reverses impotence or erectile dysfunction in some men and also reverses infertility and frigidity in some women.

EGGS

Eggs represent the ultimate protein. The protein is biologically first class. It has all the essential vitamins. Eggs is uniquely rich in the mineral "zinc" which has recently been reappraised as one of the most important nutrients necessary for growth in children. Eggs are therefore an invaluable food items for growing children, pregnant women and lactating mothers – hence, its strategic place or permanent membership in TABS. An average of 1-2 eggs per day is the acceptable for life-long vitality.Now that cholesterol is no more seen as an enemy but a friend,one can take on average 6-12 eggs a day without ill-effect.

From the economic point of view, eggs may seem expensive but they are very nourishing and have little waste products. Eggs supply a wide range of minerals and vitamins not easily available in other foods.

To make a hard-boiled egg: place the egg in a small pot with water to cover it and bring it to the boil and then continue to boil for 7-10 minutes. Then remove from the fire and cool it quickly by putting it in cool water. Eggs are best eaten boiled. Fried eggs have too much oil/fats. Raw eggs often transmit diseases like typhoid fever, therefore should be avoided as much as possible.

FISH

Fish constitutes a good source of protein, potassium, niacin, vitamin B_{12}, biotin and iodine.

Its sodium and potassium contents are well balanced compared to beef. Fish is therefore recommended for people with high blood pressure and those who want to prevent it.

Recent research has shown that regular consumption of fish and fish oils tends to lower high blood pressure. Fish is therefore highly recommended for daily consumption by patients with hypertension and those predisposed to getting it. The iodine in sea fish and oil helps to improve the complexion and general health of the skin. This is especially true for ladies who want to have young and healthy skin, they should eat fish regularly. Fish should be eaten boiled as in fresh fish pepper soup. Fried fish is harmful and should be avoided. Other acceptable methods of cooking fish are to steam, bake or grill the fish but never fry please.

It is also relevant to mention here that it is extremely important to know the source of the fish one eats. This is because fish from polluted waters of developed countries carry harmful pollutants like mercury especially fish from waters in which toxic chemical wastes have been dumped. Typical examples of polluted water would include lagoons and shore waters of developed countries. Fish imported from around Australia, New Zealand and Iceland is generally safer to eat than those from Northern Atlantic ocean and the Pacific ocean in general.

GRAPEFRUIT

This is highly recommended for its very high potassium content. It is also a very rich source of vitamin C. Being a low calorie fruit (50cal/half a grapefruit) grapefruit is a slimmer's delight.

Recent studies have shown that taking calcium antagonists such as Nifedipine (Adalat or Lomir) dissolved in grapefruit juice makes the drug more effective as an anti-hypertensive. This may be related to the high potassium content of grapefruit juice.

More recent work suggests that grapefruit juice suppresses testosterone production in me and therefore they should take the juice with this in mind.

GREENBEANS

Greenbeans is a decent source of fibre that should be consumed daily if possible especially to complement low-fibre foods at the table. It is best taken with brown rice at dinner. It is one of the best vegetables to eat at every meal: morning, afternoon and evening. Like grapefruit, oranges, and cucumber, it is very rich in potassium but low in sodium, making it a superb food for people with hypertension and those who want to prevent it. Green beans is also rich in magnesium, vitamin A and folic acid. It is to be regarded as a permanent member at every meal of the life-long vitality diet proposed in this book.

GROUNDNUTS

Groundnut is very rich in protein. Its proteins contains almost all the essential amino acids. Unfortunately its nutritive value is limited by the very low content of the essential amino acids lysine and methionine.

Arginine, aspartic acid and glutamic acid make up 50% of groundnut protein. The high levels of the amino acid – glutamic acid may be responsible for the high incidence of allergic reactions like migraine experienced by a large number of individuals who eat groundnuts. Indeed, it is thought that this amino acid may cause significant rise in blood pressure in susceptible individuals. Based on this, it is recommended that persons with high blood pressure and those predisposed to getting high blood pressure should avoid groundnuts and its oil as much as possible. This will mean avoiding deep fried foods cooked in groundnut oil as well as the popular "SUYA" meat roasted with groundnut oil. This may appear unassailable, but the reward of such self-control will be found to immeasurably outweigh any pleasure derived from eating these unhealthy snacks.

Eating badly stored fungus-infected groundnuts is thought to predispose one to getting cancer of the liver later in life. It is therefore recommended, that people eat only fresh groundnuts if necessary in order to avoid poisonous moulds in stored groundnuts.

Groundnuts have also been shown to be goitrogenic. It is therefore not recommended for regular consumption especially for persons with blood group O. The loss of libido attributed to groundnut oil may be due to the goitrogenic-like substances like gossypol. Recently, groundnut and its oil have been shown to be unhealthy for the heart when consumed regularly over a long period.

GUAVA

Guava is the richest source of vitamin C in our environment followed by red sweet pepper. It is also very rich in vitamin A. Like most fruits, it is also a great source of fibre. Guava is therefore highly recommended for daily consumption, especially when in season. The rumor that guava seeds are likely to block the human appendix and cause appendicitis is unfortunate and baseless. If anything, guava more than likely works to prevent appendicitis through its high fibre content.

GUINEACORN

Guinea corn used to be the staple crop of people living in the Northern parts of Nigeria. But over the last few decades or so, maize has gradually overtaken guineacorn as the staple diet of most average families in the country. This is most unfortunate because maize is nutritionally inferior to guinea corn. The red variety of guinea corn is to be preferred because of its rich content of iron, riboflavin, tryptophan and phosphorus.

Guinea corn has adequate and well balanced protein content as well as a high iron and calcium content. It is however, low in the amino acids methionine, cystine, tryptophan, and histidine but rich in leucine and glutamic acid. Guinea corn has lower vitamin A content compared to maize. It is a recommended cereal for weaning diets in babies because of its high iron and calcium contents.

HONEY

Honey contains over eighty substances (very close to the 91 needed to make man live interminably without disease) important for human nutrition such as glucose, many trace elements, fermentation products, organic acids, minerals, hormones, antibiotics and pollen which gives honey both its nutritional and therapeutic values for the very young and very old. For good health however, not more than one quarter (¼) of a cup of honey or 4 tablespoonfuls should be taken daily. Just a small medicinal quantity is required. About 1 tablespoonful of honey in the morning and 1 teaspoonful at night is all that is required. The dose is best taken on an empty stomach before morning workout: 2 hours before breakfast or 2 hours after evening meal. Honey is very good for the heart, especially, in the elderly. Honey taken in such "medicinal" quantities cannot harm but any larger quantity can be harmful due to its high sugar content.

Honey warmed and spread over the face helps nourish and soften skin. A teaspoonful of honey in hot milk or water before bed induces deep sleep.

IRISH POTATO

Irish potato is classically a carbohydrate that is unusually rich in potassium for a root crop. Irish potato is also rich in magnesium, copper, zinc, niacin and vitamins B_1, B_2, B_3, B_5, B_6, C, E, K, and folic acid. But particularly, fresh or raw potato is a high calorie food (125cal/potato) and is low in fiber. It should be eaten only sparingly by those who care about their weight and general health. It is healthier to eat it roasted than fried. Yet it can also be eaten boiled and mashed.

LENTILS

Lentils is a good source of protein and fibre. It is also a low calorie food (50Cal/0.28g). Lentils are rich in potassium, iron, zinc niacin and pantothenic acid – the so-called "longevity or confidence vitamin".

LETTUCE

This is very low calorie vegetable (10cal/cup). It is a perfect food for slimmers and those who care about their weight. It is a rich source of fibre. It should therefore be consumed regularly for life-long vitality and health.

Lettuce is one of the most common vegetables that are available almost all year round. It is also quite cheap and easy to grow. However, lettuce is one the most contaminated of vegetables because of its exposure to environmental pollutants during growth and harvesting.

LIME

Lime, like most citrus fruits is a good source of vitamin C, but not as good as orange. It contains 65cals/cup of its juice. It's better taken by squeezing into mineral drinks or spring water.

LIVER

Liver is the storage organ of most mammals. It is therefore no surprise that it contains virtually all minerals and vitamins. It should be eaten regularly for its rich source of vitamins, especially, vitamin B_{12} which is not so easily found in other foods. Indeed, there is no plant food that is a good source of vitamin B_{12} for man. This is the reason why vegetarians sometimes become deficient in this all important vitamin.

Liver is also rich in Vitamin A and iron. The iron in liver is more readily available for absorption than iron in cereals because liver has no phytates that interfere with the absorption of iron.

LOCUST BEAN SEED (Dadawa)

Locust bean seed is unique among all plant foods because of its very high calcium and phosphorus content. When used in large enough quantity, it could very well be substituted for animal source of calcium. Weight for weight, it is the richest source of iron in our environment followed by millet, baobab leaves and okra.

Locust bean seed or dadawa is the traditional seasoning agent in most local communities in Nigeria. In view of the intolerably high salt content in sodium monoglutamate (MSG), it is wise to avoid it in favour of locust bean seed which is natural and without any preservatives. It could be prepared together with fermented soya beans flour to give it delicious aroma,similar to or better than MSG!

A study published in Dakar Medical Journal said that regular consumption of locust beans could lower blood pressure, high blood sugar and high cholesterol level as well as prevent stroke. The journal noted that locust beans contain high level of unsaturated fatty acid (oleic acid) that prevents breast cancer and boosts high density lipoprotein (HDL or good cholesterol). At the same time, locust beans lower cholesterol and low density lipoprotein (LDL or bad cholesterol).

MAIZE

Maize is richer in oil than any other cereal. The oil is polyunsaturated (PUFA). Maize is also very high in calorie. It is richer in vitamin A than any other cereal (especially the yellow variety of maize). It is also rich in chlorine and sulphur.

As a food, however, maize is very severely limited by the composition of its main protein fraction, zein, which contains only a small amount of the essential amino acids, lysine and tryptophan. This severe deficiency of tryptophan coupled with a relative shortage of nicotinic acid, predisposes most maize eaters to the disease called "pellagra". Moreover, the deficiency of lysine and tryptophan means that maize as a staple food cannot support the growth of children well. Maize milling, which is common in certain areas, further impoverishes the maize by removing its vitamin B complex group of vitamins. Children fed on maize pap as a weaning diet are more likely to get kwashiorkor than those fed on guineacorn. The only way to improve the biological value of maize protein is by adding milk to the maize food. But because most people cannot afford milk, it is better to avoid maize as staple food. This will go a long way to reduce the high incidence of childhood malnutrition in our society. We have actually embarked on a campaign nationally to discourage families from subsisting on maize. They should instead make guineacorn or millet their staple food. If one must eat maize, the food must be taken along with milk or other cereals like wheat. Maize as staple food predisposes entire communities to becoming obese as observed in South African women who subsist on "mealie" as their staple food. Maize slows down body metabolism thereby causing fattening especially in women. Maize also favours formation of fat in the body. From personal experience, when my obese patients stopped eating maize, their weight dropped dramatically, particularly those whose blood group is not compatible with maize. This is especially true for blood group O persons.

Maize, therefore, should be cultivated solely for its polyunsaturated oil and possibly for animal feeds; as is the practice in developed societies. Maize oil contains linoleic acid and because of its omega-6 (PUFA), it is highly pro-inflammatory meaning that it can cause or aggravate inflammatory diseases like arthritis, heart disease and stroke.

Further evidence that supports the theory that guinea corn, with its high iron and calcium content is superior to maize comes from the animal kingdom. Veterinarians have discovered that puppies fed on maize meals tended to have weak bones compared to those fed on guinea corn.

The association of pellagra with maize is due to the absence of tryptophan in the maize protein, zein, and to its nicotinic acid being unabsorbed unless the maize is treated with lime.

MANGO

This fruit is a rich source of vitamin A and C as well as folic acid. It contains 55 calories/cup of its juice. It may be consumed liberally without much ill-effect when in season. It is touted to be an anti-diabetic.

MARGARINE

This is made out of vegetable oils. It also has high trans-fat oil content. It is therefore a most unhealthy food and not suitable for human consumption. It is in fact best avoided.

NATURAL BUTTER (FULANI BUTTER)

This is the fat made from cow's milk. It is highly saturated but because it is natural butter, it can be eaten sparingly as a flavor only; especially if added to Thomas Affi's Breafast Salad (TABS) where it improves absorption of vitamins,and other nutrients by a factor of10.

MELON SEED (EGUSI)

Melon seed is a very popular soup item in Nigerian. It is at the same time rich in protein. The protein is biologically of high quality. Melon seed also contains a fair amount of minerals such as phosphorus, magnesium and potassium. It is also a good source of vitamins A, D and E. Its oil is very good because it is polyunsaturated. It is rich in fibre as well.

Given the above outstanding nutrient composition, melon seed is highly recommended for life-long vitality. It can be consumed daily without ill-effects. In view of its very low sodium content, it is a perfect food for persons with hypertension and those who want to prevent it. It is also good for those on salt-restricted diets. The only minor problem with melon seed is that because of its very high fat content, its regular consumption often exacerbates pimples in susceptible persons.

MILK

Milk is a first class protein containing all the essential amino acids necessary for the growth of children. The milk bottle (not the feeding bottle) should be a child's best friend.

Milk is a low calorie food (80cal/cup). It is one of the richest sources of the rare vitamin B_2 (riboflavin). Exposure of milk to sunlight, however, destroys its vitamin B_2 content. So it is better to store milk in paper bags than in transparent bottles.

Milk contains calcium, potassium, biotin, zinc, magnesium vitamin B_{12} and pantothenic acid. Enriched skimmed milk further contains vitamin A and D.

It is better to drink skimmed milk always because of its low fat content. It is recommended to slimmers and all who care about their weight except for blood Groups O and A persons who must avoid milk completely.

To make liquid milk from powdered skimmed milk, one should add one cup of powdered milk to four cups of water and stir. To make a glass of milk, add 2 tablespoons of the powdered milk to a glass of water and stir.

Although milk is a perfect food for growing children, pregnant women and lactating mothers, it is most unhealthy for adults in view of its high salt content. Milk and milk products should be taken only sparingly if at all.

MILLET

Millet is classified as a carbohydrate but is fairly rich in protein. It is often neglected in western countries but is rich in phosphorus, magnesium, silicon, fluorine, manganese and vitamins A and B. Like guineacorn, it is fairly rich in calcium and iron. It is, however, inferior to guinea corn but superior to acha in its nutrient profile. In fact, millet is the second richest source of iron in our environment. It is used in "fura da nono" milk. Here again, tradition has been proved right by science. However, blood group O persons should eat millet sparingly because of its goitrogenic properties.

It is an excellent food for people suffering from weakness, nervous depression, or mental fatigue.

Being well supplied with vitamin A, millet has a high reputation for preventing miscarriage, correcting vitamin deficiencies in pregnant women and strengthening the body's natural defenses.

MUSHROOM

This is a very good source of fibre. It is rich in potassium, niacin, and pantothenic acid. It is a low calorie food containing only about 20cal/cup. But because there are poisonous varieties that are difficult to distinguish from non-poisonous types, one should only eat them when one is absolutely certain they are safe. Blood group O persons are to avoid mushroom as much as possible.

ONION (Longevity Spice)

Onion contains a potent germicide called acrolein that helps keep the mouth clean and odour-free. In large quantities, it is thought to lower serum cholesterol as well as bring down high blood pressure. It is also thought to lower the risk of certain cancers of the gut and is the naturopeutic mainstay for the treatment of asthma.

Onion is a good source of vitamin C and potassium. It should be eaten every morning (TABS). To reduce the pungency of onion, I usually heat it briefly in oil before eating. This routine leaves one's breath clean and fresh all day long.

Out of 100 centenarians interviewed in an American study, the only common practice amongst them was regular consumption of large amount of onions. It has been tagged the "longevity spice". The antimicrobial acrolein, found in onions has been shown to be the metabolic product of the antimitotic agent, cyclophosphamide. Whether or not the health promoting property of onions is attributed to it is not yet known for sure. Some people attribute it to its flavonoid content but this is yet to be proved unequivocally. An Italian man who had lived to over one hundred years had attributed his longevity to the practice of eating one whole onion every day without fail. I personally consume one small whole onion at breast and at dinner.It makes me sleep like a baby and wake up feeling like a blue

ORANGE

This fruit is literally a health package that is recommended as one of the major pillars of the life-long vitality diet. Orange is one of the best sources of vitamin C. It is also rich in potassium and very low in sodium. It is in fact recommended for the prevention and treatment of potassium deficiency along with banana resulting from the use of potassium-wasting drugs called diuretics.

Given its superb mineral and vitamin profile, orange is highly recommended for daily consumption by those who are hypertensive and also for those who want to prevent hypertension.

To get maximum benefit from an orange, it should be eaten whole except for the outer peals. The soft juice-bearing tissues contain another vitamin called biotin which is very important for health and vitality. This vitamin is often called vitamin H or coenzyme R.

PALM OIL

Palm oil is the most popular culinary oil in Nigeria. Unfortunately, most people do not know that it is moderately saturated and should be consumed only sparingly if at all by all persons who aspire to life-long vitality. It is unhealthy for the heart and it predisposes persons with chronic liver disease (especially in HBSAg +ve) to developing cancer of the liver.It also causes (rickets) in children because it prevents calcium absorption.

PAWPAW

This is a low-calorie fruit (55cal/fruit). It is very rich in vitamins A and C. It is also rich in potassium. It is highly recommended for life-long vitality and health.

The whole plant is beneficial. The leaves can be used to tenderise meat by boiling the meat wrapped in pawpaw leaves. The fresh leaves can be used for dressing infected wounds and ulcers. If unripe pawpaw is cut into cubes and put into a bottle with water and allowed to stand for one week the resultant concoction when taken in shots three times daily is very effective for controlling the symptoms of dyspepsia, peptic ulcer and severe acute arthritis. A little olive oil added to the concoction will prevent it from going bad for weeks. Eating a handful of pawpaw seeds with lime juice is good for liver disease patients.

PEPPER

The sweet bell pepper is a low calorie fruit (15cal/pod). It is fairly rich in potassium as well as vitamin A and C. Red sweet pepper is one of the richest sources of vitamin C in our environment.

The sweet green variety of pepper is rich in vitamin P: the anti-stroke vitamin. It is best eaten raw along with tomatoes before meals as appetizers (TABS).

Cayenne pepper is an excellent cardiovascular booster that should be consumed daily with green tea.

PINEAPPLE

Pineapple is a low calorie fruit. It is a fairly good source of vitamin A and C and manganese.

PLANTAIN

Plantain is a very rich source of carbohydrate. It is also a rich source of potassium and a fair source of calcium and iron. Plantain is also rich in vitamin B_1, B_3, B_6, pantothenic acid, niacin and ascorbic acid (vitamin C). It is however, low in fibre.

With such a healthy mineral and vitamin profile, plantain is recommended for life-long vitality. It is accordingly highly recommended for regular consumption except for blood Group O persons.

It is best prepared by boiling it in-skin and eaten with stew at breakfast.

PORK

Pork is a good source of zinc and is one of the richest sources of thiamine and vitamin B_{12} as well as the mineral selenium.

Unfortunately, its saturated fat levels are very high and therefore must be eaten only sparingly, and even then, one must eat only truly lean pork with no visible fat whatsoever.

Bacon is a product of pork, but because of its high salt content it is only mentioned to be condemned. It should be avoided at all cost because of its high fat and high salt content.

QUAKER OATS "Excellent For Diabetics"

Quaker oats is rich in manganese, iron, calcium and magnesium. It contains a stimulating substance similar to growth hormones. Oats act as an accelerator of thyroid function in the body. They stimulate and accelerate metabolism. They contain a hormone similar to folliculin that is said to combat sterility and impotence. Oatmeal at breakfast or dinner would be very great for all Nigerians especially diabetics.

RAISINS

Raisin is a good source of iron, potassium and magnesium.

RICE

Brown rice, when not polished is a rich source of vitamin B complex, especially, vitamin B_1. It is also rich in protein and oils.

Polishing (that is the process of turning brown rice into white) removes the brown coating as well as the germ of rice seed, which contains almost all the vitamins in rice. This makes polished (white) rice highly inferior to brown rice. We must therefore avoid eating white rice and stick to brown, locally milled rice always.

The best method of cooking brown rice is to use a ratio of one cup of rice to 2 cups of cold water add a teaspoonful of olive oil then bring to boil till the water dries up. The olive oil helps to prevent the rice grains from sticking together. There is no need whatsoever to bring down the rice to wash it and later replace it on fire just to make it look white. This is stack ignorance and unwise practice that robs the food of most of its vitamins and minerals. One fallacy I picked up recently listening to a University don was that he only ate snow-white rice or Uncle Ben's rice, because he believes locally milled brown rice contain little stones which could give him appendicitis. Nothing could be further from the truth! It is actually the regular consumption of white, highly processed rice that is likely to cause appendicitis because it has little or no fibre. Fibre in brown rice actually protects against appendicitis as I mentioned earlier. To carry the argument further, my Consultant Surgeon and teacher, who worked for a long time in a mission hospital in Jos, Plateau State of Nigeria used to say that whenever a patient presented with abdominal pain, the first thing he wanted to know was whether or not the patient could speak English. If he or she could not speak English, the diagnosis was unlikely to be appendicitis. It is the so-called elites who eat highly processed food with little or no fibre that get appendicitis and not the local folks who cannot afford highly polished Uncle Ben's rice. So to avoid appendicitis, and many other diseases (including heart disease), stick to brown local rice with lots of vegetables and fruits every day.

SALT

There are two types of salt: refined table salt and unrefined sea salt. Refined salt is the salt sold in the market, while sea salt is sold as deep sea salt in supplements.

Refined salt is toxic to the body and triggers many degenerative diseases including hypertension, diabetes, stroke, arthritis, glaucoma, cancer, kidney failure and heart disease.

Iodine salt is fortified with potassium iodate which is heat sensitive. When it is exposed to sunlight or heat for a long time as is the case in our markets, and during cooking the iodine escapes leaving ordinary salt that is unwholesome and even toxic. You should rely on sea salt and not iodinated salt for regular seasoning of family meals. It should be made an indispensable part of a healthy diet. The benefits of sea salt include:

a.   Carries nutrients to cells.

b.   Regulates blood pressure and blood volume to heat hypertension and leg edema.

c.   Facilitates digestion of food and absorption of nutrients.

d.   Keeps the body in electrolyte harmony and balance.

The difference between refined table salt and sea salt is in their content of trace mineral composition. While refined table salt contains 99% sodium chloride with 1% iodine, unrefined salt contains 100% macro trace elements such as; 84% sodium chloride, 14% magnesium, calcium and potassium and the remaining 2% is made up of other essential elements.

While refined table salt causes elevation of blood pressure, unrefined sea salt lowers high blood pressure and normalizes over time. It restores good digestion and corrects allergies and skin diseases. It restores good digestion especially in the elderly. Unrefined salt also eliminates excess sodium form the body and prevents fluid accumulation in idiopathic leg swelling of middle-age.

Other benefits of unrefined sea salt include: prevention of the body against chronic illnesses, mild chronic dehydration (MCD), normalizing hormonal balance in the body and controls hypertension, diabetes mellitus and muscle strength and tone.

The recommended sea salt for the family includes Brittany Sea Salt mined from Gibraltar and Himalayan salt.

SEAFOODS

The common seafoods include crabs, kelp, dulce, oyster, shrimps, lobsters, fish, periwinkles and crayfish. They are all very good sources of iron and magnesium. They are fairly low in calorie. Moreover, because of their high level of salt content which far outstrips their potassium content, sea foods are unsuitable for regular consumption except for kelp, which is highly recommended for daily consumption for its iodine and other essential mineral content. This is particularly true for blood group O persons.

The iodine content of sea foods help maintain healthy, clear skin and complexion. Their high phosphoric and zinc content is responsible for their legendary aphrodisiac qualities.

SOFTDRINKS

Most soft drinks contain high amounts of sugar and salt. They contain an average of 5-7 cubes of white sugar per bottle. They are literally "calories in the nude". They should be avoided as much as possible. Ordinary water is best for quenching thirst. Moreover, soft drinks contain colouring agents, preservatives and additives, some of which are harmful to the body. Soft drinks in excess tend to depress sexual potency and it is also a factor in the development of chronic liver disease in susceptible persons. They should be avoided like the plague.

SESAME (Beniseed)

Weight for weight, beniseed is the richest source of phosphorus in our environment. It is also very rich in calcium, iron, zinc proteins, amino acids, vitamin B_{12} and healthy fat.

Regular consumption of sesame seeds favours endocrine balance in the body that leads to longevity and strength (sexual).

In view of the very high phosphoric content, beniseed has been associated with extraordinary aphrodisiac properties. Indeed, the regular consumption of beniseed soup with pounded yam (which is rich in the vitality amino acid arginine) is said to be the secret behind the legendary virility of our brothers from Benue State of Nigeria. For this reason beniseed has been made a permanent member of the TABS.

Beniseed is also a very rich source of iron which is very good for growing children and lactating mothers. In Eggon culture, women who have delivered babies are made to eat lots of beniseed soup for the first seven days. This is another case where science has proved culture right.

SOYABEANS

Soyabeans is the only commonly available food item of plant origin that is rich in all essential amino acids.

Soyabean is a good source of thiamine, riboflavin and niacin. It is also fairly rich source of fibre.

Before soya beans is prepared into any dish for human consumption, however, it must be thoroughly roasted at 100 degrees Centigrade for about 30 minutes to destroy certain toxic alkaloids present in the seeds. In view of the high cost of animal protein that is currently beyond the reach of most families in the country, soyabeans is a good substitute for animal protein for family health.

Moreover, it has also been found to be goitrogenic especially for blood group O persons. It is not to be eaten regularly, especially for men who are overweight or obese because of its oestrogenic effects.

Soyabean oil in the market may not be entirely safe because it is produced through the process called "solvent extraction" by mixing it with inorganic hydrocarbon solvent, whose residual hydrocarbon may prove potentially harmful if not properly extracted. This may be contribution for the high incidence of cancer linked to consumption of vegetable oils in industrial countries. On the other hand only vegetable oils produced by compression extraction such as extra virgin olive oil, atili oil and avocado oil are healthy oils recommended for consumption. To worsen matters, most soyabean oils in the market are produced from genetically modified (GMO) crops for which the jury is still not yet out on their safety.

SPINACH

Spinach is a nutrient all-rounder. It is particularly rich in calcium, iron and fibre. Its potassium and sodium contents are in a balanced state. It is also rich in magnesium. Spinach is rich in vitamins A, C and folic acid and contains a significant amount of iodine. It has high antioxidant power that works to prevent or reverse age-related macular degeneration.

It is a low calorie food (40cal/cup) is very cheap and available year round. Spinach should therefore be consumed daily for life-long vitality. It is a "daily must" for health! Hence, its strategic place in TABS.

It is noteworthy to mention that some species of spinach with tiny leaves have been found to have strong goitrogenic properties responsible for endemic goiter in certain communities on the Jos Plateau. One should therefore eat only spinach that has large foliage.

SUGARCANE

Sugar cane is a high carbohydrate food because of its very high sugar content from which white sugar is obtained. Sugar cane is a rich source of vanadium and potassium. Refining sugarcane into white sugar removes all of these nutrients and leaves only unhealthy white sugar. It is thought that too much sugarcane consumption leads to cataract due to deposition of insoluble sugar complexes in the lens of the eyes. The immature growing ends of sugarcanes are very poisonous because of their cyanogenic content. Immature ends of sugar cane should not be eaten at all.

SWEET POTATO

This is nutritional dynamite that has long been neglected. It should form the cornerstone of family nutrition across the country. Polynesians in the Pacific Ocean who subsist on sweet potatoes grow tall, strong and energetic.

Sweet potato is a most wholesome food item which has been ignorantly neglected for a long time. Nutritionally, it is superior to Irish potato in many respects. It is unique in having a very high level of vitamin E – the so-called "anti-ageing" vitamin. It also contains more vitamins A and C than Irish potato. More important the vitamin C in sweet potato is not destroyed by cooking temperature.

Unlike most root crops, sweet potato is a good source of fibre. The protein of sweet potato has a high biological value and its carbohydrate is highly digestible. For life-long vitality therefore, it is strongly recommended for regular consumption (TABS). It should be boiled in-skin and eaten whole for maximum nutritional benefits of the nutrients as well as its fibre content. According to Benjamin Walker, "A Papua Guinean tribe with great physique, strength and stamina have thrived for centuries on a diet that consists almost exclusively of sweet potatoes".

BLACK TREACLE

This is also known as molasses. It is a by-product of the processing of sugar cane to white sugar. It is an excellent source of the B vitamins, iron, calcium and trace minerals. It should be used as a substitute for sugar in all homes. It is also rich in inositol, the B vitamin said to prevent premature greying of hair when taken together with folic acid, PABA, Brewer's yeast and liver.

Black treacle should replace white sugar as sweetener for the whole family. The very high iron and calcium contents in treacle are particularly important for growing children, pregnant women, and lactating mothers. Black treacle is also very rich in magnesium – the health promoting mineral.

COMPOSITION OF BLACK TREACLE AND GOLDEN SYRUP
(Per 100g)

	Units	Black Treacle	Golden Syrup
Protein	(g)	1.06	0.35
Fat	-	Nil	Nil
Carbohydrate	(g)	67.4	78.0
Calcium	(mg)	495.0	26.0
Iron	(mg)	9.2	1.4
Energy	(MJ)	1.07	1.24
Potassium	(mg)	1,550.00	?

TURKEY

The turkey meat contains more protein and fewer calories (114cal/0.28) than chicken. It is also rich in potassium, magnesium, phosphorus, iron, niacin, biotin and pantothenic acid. Turkey also has one and a half times the zinc content of chicken. It is therefore a superb meat to eat when available and if not contraindicated by blood group.

WATERMELON

This is a very low calorie food (12cal/0.37g). It is a good filler for slimmers. It contains potassium and pantothenic acid. It is recommended for daily consumption. It is also a rich source of iron.

WHEAT

Wheat is a superb complex carbohydrate that is low in calorie and also in sodium. It is a superb source of fibre, except where it is contraindicated for several blood groups.

Its protein quality is of low biological value because it is deficient in amino acids lysine and methionine. Wheat is however, a rich source of minerals and vitamins especially vitamin E. Refining of wheat into white flour removes almost all its nutrients. The process of refinement which is used to make white bread, biscuits and other junk food removes almost all nutrients. It is therefore wise to eat brown bread rather than white bread. Moreover, white bread has even higher salt content.

Wheat-germ is one of the best sources of vitamin E, zinc, iron and all the B vitamins. Half a cup of wheat germ contains four times as much proteins found in an egg.

YAM

Compared to cassava, yam has a fairly high amount of protein. The protein in yam is high in arginine, leucine and valine but low in methionine, histidine, cystine and tryptophan. Yam is also rich in vitamin A and it is a fairly good source of minerals and vitamin B complex. However, because of its low fibre content it should be eaten with lots of fibre-rich vegetables (vegetable soup) and fruits. Since it is a starchy root carbohydrate, it is good to eat it boiled in the morning at breakfast for steady release of energy from morning to afternoon. This helps people keep awake, alert and attentive right through the morning till lunch time. This practice of eating boiled starchy root carbohydrate in the morning obviates the need for harmful cups of tea or coffee to keep one alert in the office.

The high arginine content of yam helps maintain virility and sexual potency in yam consumers. The legendary virility and the sexuality in those who eat lots of yam may be attributed to this amino acid content of yam.

Recent work on obesity has shown that eating fresh starchy root carbohydrates (pounded yam, sweet potatoes, and cocoyam) in the morning helps obese persons lose weight. The reason behind this is not quite well understood. It is thought that starchy root carbohydrate tends to create a feeling of fullness that prevents the obese person from eating between meals otherwise highly fattening foods. Another reason is the fact that starchy roots like yam, cocoyam, and sweet potatoes have low calorie per gram compared to cereals. However, the calorie content of these starchy root tubers in root tubers is increased by 300% (because of removal of moisture when they are dried and made into powdered forms like Amala (yam) and fufu/alibo (cassava). These powdered forms of starchy tubers are very high calorie foods per gram that should be avoided by all who want to avoid obesity and ill-health.

YEAST (Brewer's)

Yeast, especially powdered Brewer's yeast, occupies a very unique place in the life-long vitality diet for several reasons. Yeast contains about 16 vitamins and minerals in their natural state. It is very rich in certain important vitamins that are otherwise difficult to get from common African foods. These include riboflavin, pantothenic acid, Vitamin B_6, Vitamin B_{12} and Vitamin E. A daily dose of yeast powder, therefore, supplies more than the daily requirements of these vital elements of nutrition in their near-ideal state.

Yeast can be taken simply by adding a tablespoonful of the powder to a glass of fruit juice or to any dish for that matter. Powdered Brewer's yeast is better than proprietary yeast tablets dispensed in hospital pharmacies because one may need to take 10-15 tablets of yeast to attain the efficacy of 1 tablespoonful.

A tin of Brewer's yeast should therefore supplant the salt-bottle at the family dining table for life-long vitality for the whole family.

To acquire the recommended daily allowance of pantothenic acid, Vitamin B_6 and vitamin B_{12} which are otherwise difficult to get from normal African diets, one should take about 2 tablespoonfuls of Brewer's yeast (one each at breakfast and lunch) every day for lifelong vitality and health.

YOGHURT

Yoghurt is a superfood (for those whose blood group is compatible with it) because it contains certain bacteria that manufacture generous amounts of the B group of vitamins in the digestive tract. Yogurt is particularly recommended for the health of the sex glands. The legendary virility of Bulgarian men is attributed to their regular consumption of yoghurt.

The sour milk (nono) sold by Fulani women is a form of yoghurt. Research work in India has discovered that cow's milk similar to (nono) is loaded with harmful substances called "aflatoxin" which has been linked to diseases of the liver including cancer. To my knowledge, no such research has been done in Nigeria.

JUNK FOODS AND HEALTH

Parents who are hooked on junk foods are likely to give their offsprings diabetes mellitus. This was first demonstrated in rats and through retrospective studies that has been extrapolated to humans. This may explain the sudden rise in juvenile type diabetes which was rare in Nigeria before now. According to Marilyn and Sarah, junk food produces junk children.

American researchers have discovered that junk foods programmed the human brain to crave even more sugar, salt and fat laden food. Such craving is as addictive as heroine and tobacco smoking. That is why some people find it extremely difficult to break away from junk foods despite the overwhelming evidence and statistics to show that junk foods cause obesity, destroys immunity and quality of life and eventually kills sooner or later. Once the condition starts, it is perpetuated by compulsive overeating habits similar to compulsive drug use in drug addicts.

This sugar addiction makes it extremely difficult for obese persons to lose weight. To succeed in losing weight in this group, it is crucial to start by breaking the sugar addiction first using avocado sugar extract and other appetite suppressants.

Fast foods are foods that are cooked in oil and sold at the roadside or streets. They include things like hamburger, pastries, French fried chips, fried fish, pizza, kosai, akara, masa, fried plantain, and so on.

The process of cooking fast foods involves deep frying in oils and worse, the repeated reusing of the oil over and over to cook more foods. The process of reusing oils is the most harmful of all culinary practices because it encourages the formation of substances that cause cancer, first in the cooks who inhale the toxic fumes and also in those who buy the food and eat them. In addition to cancer, excessive consumption of fried foods is linked with diseases of the heart and blood vessels – the number one killer of humanity the world over.

TREE NUTS/SEEDS

For total health and life-long vibrancy, it is highly recommended that a person eats nuts/seeds. They should always be eaten raw (never cooked or roasted). Cooking or roasting renders them acidic, and destroys enzymes and denatures their amino acids (e.g. arginine) present in them. The best way of eating almonds and sesame seeds, therefore, is to soak them in water overnight and take them (nut/seed and water) in the morning or mix it fresh with breakfast (TABS).

CHAPTER 16
WATER

(Rene Dubos)

Water, both inside and outside the human body is a great cleansing agent. It is recommended that one drinks eight glasses of water per day for optimum health. The body utilizes the water so taken to dilute impurities in the body for subsequent excretion in urine through the kidneys.

SOURCES OF WATER AND THEIR SAFETY

The various sources of potable water include: rain water, rivers and streams, spring water, ponds, pipe-born water, shallow and deep wells and boreholes;

1. Rivers and Streams

Water from streams and rivers are often highly polluted because it must have traveled over long distances passing through several human settlements, carrying sewage, industrial pollution and agricultural pollutants. They are not good for human consumption, unless properly treated.

2. Ponds and other Stagnant Waters

These sources of water are also potentially highly polluted because they receive pollution washed in from its surroundings, washed in by rains. Like water from streams and rivers, it must be properly treated before human consumption.

3. Rain Water

This may appear clean but it is loaded with atmospheric pollutants (acid rain). Moreover, as the water runs off roof tops it collects bird's droppings. It must also be well treated before drinking.

4. Shallow Well

These are wells that do not penetrate the first impervious layer of the earth's crust. They are potentially dangerous because disease germs and pollutants seep horizontally from cesspools and other sources into the well water. Water from shallow wells must not be used for drinking at all. Unfortunately, most wells in our towns and cities, particularly in our ghettos and slums fall into this category. Water from such wells must be properly boiled and then cooled before drinking every time.

5. Deep Wells and Boreholes

These provide the safest and healthiest source of water for human consumption. They are rated better than pipe-bone water in view of the fact that chemicals used for treatment of surface water (e.g. chlorine) may not be entirely safe.

6. Spring Water

Spring Water is clean if it comes from deep underground. The only precaution is to allow a chemist check the quantity of various heavy metals dissolved in the water to ensure that they are within acceptable levels for human consumption.

7. Pipe-borne Water

This is supposed to be the ultimate in potable water sourcing. The major draw-back is the ever-present risk that the water may not be properly treated because of the frequent unavailability of necessary chemicals used for treatment. In addition, the commonest chemical used for water treatment, (chlorine), has been remotely linked with certain forms of skin diseases and cancer of the bladder. This makes pipe-borne water second best (after water from deep wells and boreholes). It is best reserved for domestic washing but not for drinking or bathing because of chlorine and other treatment chemicals.

For those who really care and can afford it, it is better to boil and drink water from boreholes, spring and deep wells than drinking treated surface waters.

Finally, outside the human body, water is a very good invigorating agent. Indeed, some people ascribed some healing power to it. A cold bath in the morning tones the muscles and helps invigorate the mind and body alike through improved blood circulation to all organs. A warm bath in the evening guarantees a golden sleep at night.

WATER THERAPY

Water drinking for therapeutic purpose in the form of what is now tagged "water therapy" is an established practice that has been touted to prevent, control or ameliorate diseases like: hypertension, ulcer, diabetes mellitus, constipation, cancer and tuberculosis.

Recent work in Japan has shown that taking about six glasses of cool plain water first thing on waking up in the morning is helpful in a number of disease conditions. The water so taken helps to flush out impurities from the blood. In addition, the water helps to clean out the colon during defecation to prevent constipation. Drinking plenty of water also helps treat and or prevent diseases of the urinary tract by flushing out bacteria.

Water therapy involves drinking about 1.5 litres of water on waking before brushing, and abstaining from any food or liquid for the next 1 hour there after.

In view of the fact that the digestion of food in the stomach requires a very acidic milieu, it is not advisable to drink too much water along with food at the table. One should only drink water between meals (30 minutes before and 1 hr after) to allow for proper digestion of food and to prevent food poisoning.

Moreover, water, important as it is for optimum health, is easily the most important vehicle of disease in man. One should only drink water that is pure and free of disease causing organisms. Good drinking water should have no taste, colour and smell.

The only source of concern with water therapy is the potential for disease transmission. The chance of transmitting disease is proportional to the quantity of water taken at a time. So that to prevent catching any typhoid fever for instance, the water to be taken must be boiled and allowed to cool overnight before drinking. The most convenient and economical way of doing this is to use a large kettle especially made for that purpose. The water is boiled as soon as the evening meal is done. After boiling, the water is allowed to cool overnight.

Another very convenient method is to use a water tank that has BFSUMA filter installed so that the whole family can enjoy safe, potable water no matter the source. The BFSUMA filter is cheap and doable and therefore highly recommended for every office, or institution or village water point.

CHAPTER 17
HONEY AND HEALTH

When I travelled to Britain for the very first time in 1986 as a student, I had had in mind the secondary objective of unravelling the mystery behind the paradox of the former British Empire where a small Island country like Britain had conquered and ruled virtually the whole world; where the sun rose and set in the empire.

I was curious to know the secret behind their guts, stamina, courage, character and determination which had fostered the ambition for such stupendous accomplishment.

After sifting through numerous possibilities, honey consumption stood out as one of the most plausible reason for the unique qualities that had enabled the British bring off such monumental administrative and military exploits needed to subdue the whole world.

The above postulation that honey might have had a posititive impacton British in character conduct and drive has been amply corroborated by the following historical averments:

When Phoenician traders came to Britain in search of tin and lead during the pre-Christian era, they found enormous quantities of honey in Britain and named the Island "The Isle of Honey". Separately, the Druids also in Britain before the Christian era had called Britain, "The Honey Isle of Beli".

Furthermore, one of the pre-Christian historians, written that, "These Britons only begin to grow old at 120". Yet another wrote that the islanders consumed large quantities of honey-brew (or mead).

A little later in history, when the Romans landed in Britain, they found that all the Britons were very strong and beautiful. Even today, people from America and continental Europe go to Britain to pick marriage partners. The men are said to be attracted by the exotic beauty and character of British girls who are descendants of their ancestral heavy honey eaters.

In the Tudor days of Britain, the citizens were reputed to be robust, adventurous and strong; all these qualities were attributable to massive honey consumption. However, in the Elizabethan era, honey consumption was replaced with consumption of white sugar which I believe destroyed the character and nativity of the people and consequently led to the eventual decline and fall of the British Empire. This is similar to the role played by lead poisoning in the decline and fall of the Roman Empire.

On longevity, honey has been shown to prolong life by lowering heart rate because of its acetylcholine content. This may well be the explanation behind the legendary longevity of beekeepers all over the world. For instance, in A.D. 23, Pliny the Elder who travelled a lot in North Italy saw in the region of the River Po and the Appenines, 124 individuals who were well over a hundred, the eldest been 135years old. They were all beekeepers.

In 1950, the Russians issued a postage stamp in honour of Eicarov Mamoud Baguir-Ogly who had reached the ripe old age of 148 years. He was a beekeeper. And Thomas Parr, A British man who had lived to be 153 years, his diet was honey, cheese and wheat-germ.

When Sir Edmund Hilary reached the top of Mt. Everest, his father who was a beekeeper had remarked "It was all done on honey". Tiger Tensing who had accompanied Sir Hilary was himself a great honey eater and so were all the porters that went on the expedition with them.

This is the narrative of the stamina, courage, and discipline which honey confers on its fervent consumers.

As for the elderly, Professor Dr. E. Koch, the famous German heart specialist had advocated that honey is ideal medicine for the heart which should be taken regularly especially by those undergoing stressful situations.

And to quote Barbara Cartland once again, "Raw unprocessed honey, because of its propolis content heals the wind pipe and the respiratory apparatus through which you breathe and live; and it benefits the soul to literally give you immortality".

In conclusion, I hope this chapter has built up a strong case for our fellow citizens to learn to consume honey more; especially raw, unprocessed honey; in order to eugenically improve the quality of our people in the country to make for accelerated development and progress of our dear nation. Still on eugenics, children that are given honey from after one year of age till adolescence tend to grow up strong, disciplined, mature and of good character.

Finally, I humbly wish to draw the attention of government to the compelling imperative to encourage Nigerians to consume more honey in order to improve the quality of our children and adults alike. The honey being advocated is raw, unprocessed natural honey; possibly eaten along with the honeycomb: one tablespoonful first thing on waking every morning and one teaspoonful at bed time.

In advocating for wholesale consumption of honey for all citizens, I am not in any way anticipating our future colonization of other countries; rather my aim is to help raise a generation of Nigerians and Africans that have desirable qualities of good citizenship, who are courageous, confident, fearless, daring and adventurous. This will go a long way to help us build, not an empire of lands, but an empire of the minds necessary to bring off the much needed African renaissance.

In conclusion therefore, nothing is better for health and longevity of our citizens than to add the right proportion of honey to their food daily.

The explanation for the beneficial effects of honey may be rooted in the recent findings that have been able to show that honey acts to reduce oxidation of LDL to prevent plague formation in blood vessels thereby preventing heart disease, stroke and premature death.

CHAPTER 18
ALCOHOL AND HEALTH

Alcohol is the product of the fermentation of carbohydrates by a fungus called yeast. There are many types of alcohol that result from the fermentation of carbohydrates but the major ingredient in all alcoholic drinks is ethyl alcohol or ethanol or grain alcohol. Because alcohol supplies only calories to the body, it is considered a carbohydrate with no protein, fat, minerals, vitamins or fibre. It is therefore nutritionally the most unwholesome food item.

The ethyl alcohol is the same whether it is in brandy, ogogoro, burukutu or palmwine. The difference between the various alcoholic beverages is the percentage content of ethyl alcohol present. Beer for instance has ethyl alcohol content of about 5 –7%, wine 7% and spirits 20–40 %. Spirits such as gin, whisky and brandy contain other chemicals like enanthic ether which gives them their characteristic flavours. They also contain impurities like methyl alcohol which acts as alcohol but is even more toxic to the human body than ethyl alcohol.

Alcohol is a universal poison that is highly injurious to the body, particularly in women in which even a small amount of alcohol increases the risk of breast cancer by over 250%. Alcohol is also associated with cancer of the mouth, oesophagus, pharynx, larynx and liver.

Alcohol has been used by all human societies for a very long time mainly for social reasons, but sometimes they are used for ritual ceremonies as well. Unfortunately, it is only fairly recently that the full magnitude of the incalculable damage that alcohol does to the human body has come to be fully appreciated.

Alcohol is an absolute poison; it is toxic to virtually all tissues of the human body. It causes the greatest damage to the liver, the heart and the nervous system including the brain. Other organs seriously affected are the gastrointestinal tract, the pancreas, the eyes, the bones and the skin. The toxic effects of alcohol can be acute as well as chronic. The victim tends to live a miserable life punctuated by frequent irritating and sometimes debilitating illnesses that range from morning hangover and headaches to liver cirrhosis, heart failure and psychosis. Quite apart from these physical consequences of alcohol abuse, alcoholism affects family stability in general. Consequently, the insulted organs sooner or later fail to perform optimally resulting in premature ageing and death.

I must make myself quite clear at this juncture that I am not saying that one must never touch alcohol at all. Indeed, a little alcohol once in a while may even be good for your heart. All I am saying is that taking more than a little alcohol is definitely injurious to health. In other words, it is best to abstain, but if it proves impossible, one should restrict the intake of alcohol to social occasions only and even then, one must not take more than one bottle of beer a day. The equivalent is 2 shots of whisky, brandy, or gin.

It is noteworthy to point out once again that alcohol is more toxic to women than men. Women are less able to tolerate the toxic effects of alcohol than men. It is therefore recommended that women take much less alcohol than men. They should take only ½ of beer per day or one shot of spirit or one glass of wine only per day. This recommended amount is enough social catalyst for most occasions.

In addition to the toxic effects of alcohol, manufacturers often add certain chemicals that help preserve the ethanol in good condition for long shelf lives. These substances are often potentially harmful if consumed in large enough quantities. Examples of these additives include sulphur dioxide and sodium bisulphate. The latter is said to precipitate asthmatic attacks in susceptible individuals so that when one drinks beer or any other alcoholic drink for that matter, one is not only exposing oneself to the toxic effects of the alcohol alone but one is exposed to the toxic effects of the preservatives and impurities present in the alcohol as well. This should be enough reason to discourage any sensible person from indulging in excess alcohol.

On whether or not palm wine is safer than manufactured drinks, the answer is yes and no. Yes, perhaps because palm wine, when harvested fresh from the tree is unfermented, and devoid of harmful additives and preservatives. In this respect, palm wine is better than manufactured drinks. But the toxic effects of the ingredient, ethanol is the same, whether it is in palm wine or in manufactured drinks.

The answer to the question of whether palm wine is better than manufactured drinks can also be "NO" if it is considered that the palm wine contains certain chemicals called nitrates which is converted to nitrosamines that have been linked to cancer of the throat and oesophagus. These cancers are incidentally fairly common in our society.

A word about locally brewed alcoholic beverages: burukutu and ogogoro. The brewing of these alcoholic beverages is done in the most unhygienic settings.

Burukutu for instance, is brewed in metal drums which most likely contributes large amounts of harmful heavy metal poisoning to these drinks. Research work carried out in South Africa showed that consumption of beer brewed in metal drums resulted in high incidence of excess iron deposition in the livers of the consumers of these beverages. No such work has been done in Nigeria as far as I know but the case is likely to be the same. The end result of the deposition of large amount of iron in the liver is chronic liver disease which is often fatal.

Ogogoro on the other hand, has been shown to contain lots of impurities from the wooden containers used for distillation of this most illicit drink. The impurities are more than likely to be potently harmful, especially on the long term. A typical example of such impurities is methyl alcohol which causes blindness in the victims.

In conclusion, if one stays away from alcohol one has nothing to lose except perhaps the morning hangovers and a few alcoholic friends. On the other hand, by avoiding alcohol, one stands to gain much in life. The life rewards include a cool, sober, personality loved and trusted by family and friends, plenty quality time available to wife (husband) and children and most important, a life enriched with youthful zestfulness and sparkling vitality to the very end.

Nevertheless, if you must drink at all, then for goodness sake drink only very little at a time, and even then do it only when you really have to.

If one must drink at all, one must never drink around meal times. The practice of using table wine or beer, to wash down lunch or dinner is most unhealthy and must be condemned as one of those harmful legacies of colonialism which, unfortunately, is copied blindly by our "nouveaux riches". Wine or beer is first and foremost a "sad food" item that depresses the central nervous system, thereby robbing one of the vital forces of life. Secondly, alcohol destroys vitamin B complex in the body. Thirdly, alcohol is pure calorie in the "nude" that is no good for the body. Fourthly, beer or wine in excess goes to dilute the stomach acid thereby causing indigestion. Finally, drinking beer or wine at the table introduces a lot of water along with meals; and this which works inadvertably to cause weight gain or the so-called "beer belly" (central-obesity) that is so very lethal in the long term.

CHAPTER 19
THE CONCEPT OF AN ADEQUATE DIET

"You are what you eat"

(Victor Lindlahr)

The total number of nutrients a person needs to live without disease is 91. If one gets all the 91 nutrients, one is likely to live very long without degeneration or disease. A diet is said to be adequate when it contains food items from all classes of food in such proportions as to supply all necessary nutrients as at when needed by the body. Such a diet contains the right quantity of protein, carbohydrate, fat, minerals, vitamins and fibre. In other words a diet can be inadequate in terms of its composition, its quality as well as its quantity. For instance, an ideal diet should contain 70% starchy carbohydrate, 20% healthy fat, 10% high quality protein (70:20:10).

A typical African diet is inadequate because it often contains more than 90% carbohydrate, 5% unhealthy fat, and little or no protein (90:5:5). The diet predisposes the victim to protein-calorie malnutrition, nutritional anaemias, lowered immunity, frequent infections, vitamin deficiencies, erectile dysfunction and so on. These together lead to premature aging and shortened life expectancy. Such a diet weakens the bodily immunity and exposes it to all sorts of diseases including infection, cancers and degenerative ailments.

On the other hand, the average diet of western industrialized nations (and the more affluent members of our society) is inadequate because it contains 20% starchy carbohydrate, 40% protein, 40% fat, (20:40:40). Such diet predisposes to an even longer list of diseases: Hypertension, diabetes mellitus, autoimmune disease, peptic ulcer disease, inflammatory bowel disease, gallbladder stones, hyperlipidemia, heamorrhoids, anal fissures, colon cancer, oesophageal reflux, appendicitis and ovarian cancer etc.

The most important principle of an adequate diet therefore, is the provision of as many nutrients as possible in one meal. I shall illustrate this fundamental principle of nutrition as follows: suppose a builder wants to build a wall, he needs to have water, cement, and bricks made available to him all at once before he can set upon his job. It is no use having plenty of sand, brick and water but no cement to keep these items stuck together. It is also futile to have plenty of water, sand and cement but no bricks to build with. To build a strong wall, the mason needs all necessary items provided at once. That is how it is with nutrients and our physical body building.

EATING FOR HEALTH

What does it take to eat for health? You don't need to give up your favourite food or set up a cumbersome system of rules or calorie counting. And you don't even need to have a particular body weight to be fit. You should make eating a pleasurable and adventurous experience every time.

PRINCIPLES:

a.   Eat according to your blood group – it is fundamental.

b.   Be realistic: make small changes at a time.

c.   Be adventurous: experiment with new foods one at a time.

d.   Be flexible–avoid being rigid.

e.   Be sensible: enjoy as many foods as possible, only don't overdo it.

f.   Be active–to lose or maintain ideal weight.

GUIDELINES:

- Avoid all deep-fried foods, no matter the dainty
- Emphasize fruits, vegetables, whole grains and fat free or low-fat milk and milk products.
- Include lean meat, poultry, fish, beans, eggs, nuts and seeds.
- Eat foods that are low in salt, zero in sugar and zero in trans-fats.
- Food should be prepared and handled hygienically to keep safe.

CHALLENGES OF HEALTHFUL CHOOSING OF FOOD

- Cost
- Too much effort
- Limited know-how
- Too many people in the house
- Ill-health
- Old age

The above analogy beautifully illustrates the fundamental principle of an adequate diet: that the diet provides all the essential nutrients as at when needed. If not, the available items cannot work in isolation. This is because the human body has no facility for storage of unused protein while excess fats and oils is converted to body fat, and is not immediately available when a sudden need for energy arises.

A detailed knowledge of the nutrient composition of different food items commonly available as is necessary for one to select different food items based on their nutritional values to draw up an adequate diet. This detailed knowledge enables one to create suitable permutations of balanced and delicious meals to suit each occasion and palate at breakfast, lunch, and supper. It also enables one to know which foods to eat at each meal and which nutrients are missing in a particular meal. With this knowledge, one can make necessary arrangements to supplement one's dietary requirements with proprietary preparations of either minerals and/or vitamins.

I must emphasize strongly here that one should never make it a habit of taking proprietary vitamins and minerals indiscriminately. It is much healthier to acquire all of one's nutrients (91 of them) through eating fresh, unprocessed foods. The main reason being that natural sources of nutrients have in addition, certain yet unknown substances that assist the various known nutrients to perform their physiological functions optimally. Science has not been able to characterize these "supportive substances" just as yet. For instance, the protective effect which vitamin A confers on its consumers against certain cancers is only achieved by eating natural sources of carotene, the precursor of vitamin A. Proprietary preparations of vitamin A lack this protective effect against cancer. Indeed taking proprietary β-carotene has been linked with increased incidence of cancer of the lungs.

Another very important aspect of an adequate diet concerns the quantity of each food item consumed at a sitting. It is hopeless having all the different classes of food at one's disposal, and only to eat them in the wrong proportions. This is the problem with most of our more affluent compatriots. They eat far too much protein and fats on the erroneous conviction that they are enjoying themselves. They soon develop pot-bellies and fat lobed necks which they believe are signs of having "arrived" economically. Little do they know that these sad features of obesity herald their gradual but certain departure from the scene and certainly not "arrival" as wrongly believed.

Research has shown that animals fed purely on denaturalized diet (cooked and fast foods), had remained alive but their state of health was mediocre: a state of semi-nutrition called MESOTROPHY (malnutrition). This is the status of 80% of our citizens today. This mediocre health led to symptoms of degeneration such as falling out of teeth, chronic constipation, softening of bones and diminished physical capacity. When these animals were again fed on green vegetables, cereal, wheat-germ or Brewer's yeast, the malnutrition disappeared and some of the animals made full recovery.

The above research finding corroborates the view of some experts that the majority (80%) of human diseases are rooted in nutritional deficiencies resulting from cooked or denaturalized, processed foods. To attain optimum health, therefore, we must give up deep-rooted nutritional habits nationally as a meter of governmental policy. It will make a wide difference between a short miserable life and a long happy, productive and fulfilled life.

I shall therefore proceed to spell out the recommended quantity, quality and nature of different food groups that promote and maintain life-long health and vitality.

CARBOHYDRATES

Carbohydrates form the bulk of the food we eat every day. They include foods like yam, rice, guinea corn, millet, cassava, amala and so on. Their function in the body is to provide energy for movement as well as energy for physiological and mental work. For optimum health, starchy grains and root carbohydrate should constitute 70% of all total calories eaten in a day; too little carbohydrate can lead to energy malnutrition.

A good rule of thumb is to eat enough carbohydrates to take the edge off one's hunger. A rough and ready estimate is to eat 2 handfuls or a lump of food that is about the size of one's fist at a sitting. Any more than that is excess and unhealthy. The energy in the lump of pounded yam is enough for most people except maybe for wood hewers and ditch diggers. This rule is however not applicable for children because children are still growing and need relatively more food for the size of their bodies.

For daily vitality, carbohydrate is best eaten as unprocessed, starch, cereals and root carbohydrates. They should be eaten boiled not fried. Processed or refined carbohydrates such as wheat flour, white sugar or dried powdered starch, (amala, eba, alibo, fufu) are high calorie and should be avoided as much as possible. It is important to bear in mind that processing of root carbohydrates into flour – cassava flour (alibo, garri or fufu); yam flour (amala) renders them very unhealthy for two reasons. First the process of flour making robs those root carbohydrates of vitamins and moisture which means that weight for weight, the calorie content of these foods is increased by about 300%. This makes them highly unsuitable for people watching their weight and those who want to maintain their ideal body weight. Fufu, alibo, gari and amala are therefore high calorie foods which are inimical to long life. For longevity, therefore, it is better to eat fresh, unprocessed starchy foods (boiled root vegetables like yam, pounded yam, cocoyam, sweet potatoes, etc) direct from the farm in order to restrict calorie intake for increased lifespan.

I shall take time to explain this in more detail why avoiding refined carbohydrate (white sugar) is often the most difficult aspect of the life-long vitality diet. Most people cannot believe that something so sweet and apparently harmless as sugar should be the bane of good nutrition. But lo and behold it is true and white sugar is now tagged "universal poison" by nutritionists.

When starchy carbohydrates like grains, yam, cocoyam, potato, cassava are eaten, the digestive enzymes in the mouth, stomach and intestines take about 1-3 hours to work on them to reduce them into small molecules that can be absorbed into the blood and taken to various places for release of energy in the body. The most important of these end products is glucose. It is, indeed, the final end-point of all carbohydrate digestion. White sugar requires little time for digestion. When it is consumed, it is promptly absorbed with little digestive activity. This leads to sudden upsurge in the level of glucose in the body. Before glucose is utilized by most organs of the body, it requires the presence of a certain chemical hormone called insulin. Insulin is manufactured in the body in the organ called pancreas. For normal physiological function, insulin is released in slow, pulsed phases. This is naturally compatible with the slow release of glucose from the digestion of starchy carbohydrates but not with refined sugar. When white sugar is eaten, it is suddenly shoved into the blood stream. This sets off a strong signal to the pancreas for it to produce correspondingly large amount of insulin to cope with the sudden upsurge in blood glucose. The insulin causes prompt reduction in blood sugar to a very low level in about 2 hours. Because the brain uses 60% of blood glucose, it is the first to manifest symptoms of low blood sugar. These include sleepiness, yawning, lack of concentration, irritability and lethargy. The usual response of the person is to quickly request for another cup of tea loaded with sugar, hoping it would liven him or her up. The situation is temporarily arrested for another half an hour or so after the cup of tea. Soon after, however, there occurs another unnatural sudden upsurge in blood sugar only to be followed by another fall, leading to hyper insulinaemia associated symptoms of low blood sugar. The person calls for another cup of tea and the vicious circle continues. If this continues for a long period (years), the situation leads to permanent hyperinsulinaemia and subsequent metabolic syndrome X, which is associated with serious diseases like hypertension, diabetes mellitus, obesity, hypercholesterolaemia and atherosclerosis, stroke and heart attacks.

As mentioned above, the repeated sudden rise and sudden fall of blood sugar produced by white sugar and junk foods, has many deleterious effects in the body. First and foremost, it produces embarrassing, irritating bouts of sleepiness and lack of concentration in office workers at a time when they need their brains most (9am-12noon). This goes a long way to affect their decision making and general joie de vivre.

A more disturbing consequence of the frequent rise and fall in blood sugar is the long term cumulative effect on blood vessels of the body leading to destruction of the vascular wall, similar to what happens in diabetes mellitus. The most susceptible vessels are those of the eyes, the kidneys and the brain. These effects have also been implicated as possible etiological factors in essential hypertension. This is because the high level of blood sugar is toxic to blood vessels and this is referred to as glucotoxicity.

Another equally serious consequence of the unnatural sudden rise and fall in blood sugar, is the long term effect on the insulin producing organ, pancreas. The frequent unnatural demand placed on the pancreas affects its physiological response pattern, so much so that it often leads to permanent damage. The end result is the dreaded disease called Type 2 diabetes mellitus.

As you can see, therefore, white sugar is not as innocuous as it would seem at first. The highs and lows in blood sugar discussed above is not restricted to pure crystalline white sugar. It applies equally well to all foods sweetened with white sugar or those which are made with refined flour "the so-called hidden sugar". They include the following: all soft drinks, biscuits, cakes, meat-pies, all baked foods, all manufactured foods, honey, sweets, chocolates, all non-alcoholic beverages. The above listed foods must be avoided for the attainment of the lofty goal of life-long vitality and longevity.

From the explanation given above, we can conveniently avoid the highs and lows of blood sugar and at the same time reap the wholesome benefits of a gradual rise and fall of blood sugar by eating starchy carbohydrates always. They are slowly digested and then slowly absorbed. This leads to a gradual rise in blood sugar that is compatible with the physiological, pulsed release of the hormone insulin from the pancreas. The result is a constant supply of glucose to the body organs (especially the brain). The person remains alert and awake to his responsibilities and carries on indefatigably till lunch time (1pm – 2pm). The TABS breakfast that provides this harmonized situation will include: high quality protein (beans/eggs/fish/lima/bambara nut) healthy oils (olive, flaxseed, avocado, atili) and garnished with sesame seeds.

Another advantage of eating starchy carbohydrate is that the effort required for chewing them before they are swallowed contributes immeasurably to the strength of teeth and their well-being. Chewing also enables digestion to start from the mouth through the effects of salivary enzymes. This reduces the work of the stomach, which is good for general health and vitality. An even more important benefit of eating starchy carbohydrate is that they stay in the stomach longer to give a feeling of satisfaction and well-being. They also help tone the stomach to make it more efficient with time.

Another important benefit of eating starchy foods is that they contain nutrients which are absent in white sugar and refined flour. These missing items include minerals, vitamins and fibre.

Examples of starchy foods include plantain, yam, brown rice, Irish potato, sweet potato, cocoyam and cassava. They are best eaten boiled, because deep frying renders them very unhealthy. If they would be fried at all, they must be stir-fried using olive oil only. Other starchy foods are guineacorn and millet.

PROTEIN

As I mentioned earlier, only growing children, pregnant women and lactating mothers need to eat protein in any quantity. Adult men and non-pregnant women need very little animal protein for optimum health. They should eat just enough to replace worn out tissues and cells of the body. This works out to a total of about 0.4-0.6g/kg body weight per day. This is about the size of a piece of meat served with a regular plate of "rice and beans" in local "mama-put" restaurants. So that the ordering of extra meat or pepper soup or goat head or even suya is to say the least wasteful much as it is very harmful.

Animal protein, especially, must be eaten sparingly for life-long vitality. With plant proteins like beans, soyabeans, groundnuts and other legumes, however, one is allowed greater liberty without much ill-effect as long as one eats them in accordance with their blood group compatibility in mind.

Protein, especially plant protein, contains minerals and vitamins that complement those in starchy carbohydrate. More protein should be taken in the morning at breakfast than at any other time for their dynamic action – this is the energy released when food which is digested in the stomach. Beans protein is the most versatile of them all. It represents the first pillar of the life-long vitality diet. It can be eaten in the form of moi moi, or just plain boiled beans garnished with beniseed and served with fresh sauce. Beans should be eaten daily for health and vitality (see box for proper cooking of beans for health and longevity).

Soak the beans overnight to remove the natural toxins in the beans and to prevent gas and flatulence. Wash the beans again and boil and throw away the water the second time before thebeans is done.

FRUITS AND VEGETABLES: The importance of fruits and vegetables cannot be over-emphasized. They constitute the backbone of the life-long vitality diet. Their extreme importance lies in their ability to supply fibre, vitamins, minerals and phyto nutrients.

In the tropics, we are blessed with all sorts of fruits and vegetables year round. We can afford to select them to please our individual whims and tastes. The most important principle is to eat some fruits and vegetables at each meal. As a rule of thumb, proteins should always be eaten first at breakfast to enable the amino acids, tryptophan and tyrosine reach the brain before carbohydrates come on the scene. This is to enable the person remain alert and calm throughout the day. After the protein, fruits should follow before the cooked starchy carbohydrates in order to dampen the harmful generalized inflammatory reaction that follows the consumption of cooked food. The vegetables are eaten last; the reason being that vegetables help to cleanse the mouth because of their high liquid content. Moreover, they need to be chewed for a longer time, which helps to further strengthen the teeth. When this is followed by good brushing 10 minutes later, using local chewing stick followed by tooth paste brushing, the result is a clean mouth that guarantees a fresh breath and shining white teeth all day long. Fruits should be eaten first in order to damn the rise in inflammatory reaction that takes place when cooked food is eaten. Moreover, fruits being sugary should not be eaten last because of dental disease.

In summary, at breakfast, one should start with protein (fish, egg, lean meat) followed by fruits, TABS and lastly, green tea plus 5 (cayenne pepper, fresh or powdered ginger, apple cider vinegar, lemon juice and cinnamon).

FRUIT JUICE

Fruits are supposed to be eaten and not juiced. Juicing fruits makes them unhealthy because it makes them get absorbed too quickly into the blood stream without much digestion. This renders them high glycaemic index foods that raise blood sugar rapidly which encourage obesity. Worst of all, commercial fruit juices are usually cooked, pasteurized, irradiated or processed in one form or the other. This makes them not only valueless but very harmful on long term.

FATS

Fats include vegetable oils, margarine, butter and animal fat. They are very important in human nutrition because they produce the feeling of satiety after meals. They are also necessary for the production of certain chemicals like the prostaglandins and hormones. Fats also enter into the structure of the cell membranes of many tissues. They are also necessary for the absorption of fat-soluble vitamins ADEK in food.

Fats are nutritionally divided into saturated and unsaturated fats. The former are harmful to the body because they are associated with premature aging of the blood vessels of the body. This could cause stroke or heart attacks.

The unsaturated fats are less likely to cause problems and are to be preferred at all times. In fact, some unsaturated fats actually lower the risk of cardiovascular diseases. Typical examples are: fish oil, olive oil, atili oil, avocado oil, flaxseed oil and coconut oil.

Most plant oils are polyunsaturated except palm oil, palm kernel and coconut oil. Most animal fats are saturated except fish oil. In fact, the regular consumption of fish oil is thought to lower blood pressure and help prolong life.

For all I have said, however, one only needs about 3-6 teaspoonful of oils per day for optimum health. Any excess above this is harmful. It is therefore, unwise to eat anything that is deep-fried or dressed in oil. Such unhealthy meals usually adorn the tables of our more affluent compatriots who, ignorantly, regard them as trademarks of status and social "arrival". But nutritionists and dietitians regard such unhealthy dishes as harbingers of slow and painful departure from the society and the world as mentioned earlier.

The nutritionally wise should view oil-rich, deep-fried foods as the height of ignorance which must be despised and shunned as much as possible.

Eating the right foods in the right combinations can actually prevent disease from taking hold in the first place. Foods, if used correctly, have the power to prevent all kinds of serious ailments, including heart disease, diabetes, cancer, arthritis, and so on and so forth.

CHAPTER 20
FOOD ADDITIVES AND PRESERVATIVES

"The first commandment of correct eating; Thou shall not poison thyself"

(Dr T.C. Fry)

The key message in this book is to encourage readers to stick to foods that are fresh, unprocessed and as much as possible avoid all refined foods. Refined foods include virtually all manufactured and imported food items. They include inter alia, biscuits, sweets, alcoholic drinks, chocolates, cakes and all breakfast cereals. Even soft drinks are not left out. They all contain certain added chemicals to keep them from spoiling over a length of time.

Although some of these chemical additives and preservatives have been declared safe for human consumption, some of them are known to be potentially harmful. For instance, most colouring agents used in the food industry are known to be potentially unsafe.

I must make it quite clear at the outset that eating these so-called "junk" foods once in a while may be unavoidable and may not indeed be exactly harmful. It is their regular consumption that can be potentially harmful due to cumulative effects. The incidence of certain harmful growths in our society today can only be reasonably explained away by the consumption of highly processed and manufactured food items containing additives and preservatives as well as genetically modified foods (GMF).

I shall do no more than list out the common additives, preservatives and colouring agents to guide the reader in the choice of junk or manufactured foods.

S/N	UNSAFE ADDITIVES AND PRESERVATIVES	FOODS CONTAINED IN
1	Colouring Agent of any kind e.g. Tartrazine, erythrosin (Blue, Green, Yellow).They can cause cancer/allergy.	All artificially coloured foods Beverages and soft drinks.
2	Artificial flavours	Breakfast cereals
3	Aspartame (causes cancer)	Gelatin, desserts
4	Brominated vegetable oil (BVO)	Soft drinks
5	Butylate Hydroxy Anise (BHA)	Chewing gum, vegetable oils

6	Butylated Hydroxytoluene (BHT)	Chewing gum, potato chips
7	Caffeine (stimulant) may cause migraines: birth defects.	Soft drinks, coffee, tea
8	Carrageenan	Ice-cream, jelly, infant formulae
9	Corn syrup	Candy, Snack foods, syrups
10	Dextrose	Soda pop, cookies
11	Hefty paraben	Beers, soft drinks
12	Hydrogenated vegetable oil (trans-fats)	Margarine
13	Invert sugar	Soft drinks
14	Monosodium glutamate (MSG) (caused destruction of brain cells in experimental animals. High sodium content can aggravate or precipitate hypertension. It can also cause "Chinese Restaurant Syndrome"	Artificial food seasonings
15	Phosphoric acid	Breakfast cereals, cheese, soft drinks
16	Propyl gallate	Vegetable oil
17	Quinine (causes birth defects, skin rashes)	Tonic water, Bitter Lemon
18	Saccharine	Diet drinks
19	Salt (causes high blood pressure)	Most processed foods, bread, crackers, biscuits, soft drinks, breakfast cereals
20	Sodium nitrate/nitrite (causes cancer)	Corned beef, Bacon, smoked fish
21	Sucrose	All sweetened foods
22	Sodium bisulfate (destroys vitamin B_1: can precipitate asthmatic attack)	Wines and beers

A careful study of the above list will convince the inveterate consumer and the most hardened skeptics that most processed, refined and manufactured food items are unwholesome for human consumption. They contain too much salt and too much sugar. They also contain additives and preservatives, the safety of which no one can guarantee.

Moreover, refined foods are highly impoverished in terms of vitamins and minerals because the process of refinement removes most of the vital nutrients. And worst of all, manufactured food items have little or no fibre – the basic substance of life-long vitality. Instead of adding to vitality and longevity, processed foods deplete the body of essential nutrients leading to compromised impoverished bodies and eventually, premature deaths.

By way of putting the last nail into the coffin of refined and manufactured foods, I have listed out below the high-salt food items that should be avoided as much as possible.

High salt foods	High salt foods
1. Bacon	11. Sardines
2.Butter (Salted)	12. Pureed Tomato
3.Many breakfast cereals	13. Tuna
4.Cheese	14. Sausage
5.Milk	15. Baking powder (bread, cakes)
6.Margarine (Salted)	16. Self-rising flour (Yeast bread)
7. Potato chips	17. Corned beef
8. Biscuits (Salted)	18. Meat-pie
9. Salted groundnuts	19. Mono sodium glutamate (MSG)
10. Salted popcorn	

NATURAL FOOD TOXINS

Although, I have vehemently written against the unwholesome consumption of manufactured foods and all foods processed in industries, it is equally important to point out here that some natural unprocessed foods straight from the farm also contain harmful toxins. Some of the common foodstuffs and their toxins include:

S/N	FOOD ITEMS	ACTIVE AGENT	REMARKS
1	Banana	5 – HT	Heart disease- Stimulates the central nervous system

2	Cheese	Tyramine	Raises blood pressure
3	Cassava	(a) Cyanide (b) Goitrogens	Causes peripheral neuropathy and diabetes; aggravate peptic ulcer Causes goiter
4	Smoked Fish (dried fish)	Nitrosamine	Liver Damage; Cancer in animals
5	Palm-wine	Nitrosamine Nitrates	Liver Damage; Cancer in animals
6	Beans	Vicine	Haemolytic anaemia (favism)
7	Sugarcane	Cyanogen (in young canes)	Cyanide poisoning
8	Tea, Coffee, cola nuts	Methyl Xanthines	(1) Destroys vitamin C in the body (2) Birth defects (3) Hypertension (4) Arrhythmias
9	Groundnuts	(a) Aflatoxin (b) Goitrogens (c) Gossypol	Linked with liver cell cancer Goiter Loss of Libido
10	Soya beans	a. Anti-growth factor b. Goitrogen c. Carcinogen d. Oestrogen	Dwarfism Goiter Cancer of the stomach Loss of Libido especially in obese men
11	Cabbage	Goitrogen	Goiter
12	Tobacco	Carcinogen	Cancer of the mouth, lungs and oesophagus
13	Spinach with (small leaves)	Goitrogen	Goiter
14	Bushmeat(smoked)	Pyrrolidine	Liver Cancer
15	Maize beer (Burukutu)	Not Known	Cancer of the oesophagus, obesity
16	Salted fish	Salt	Hypertension
17	Plantain	5 – HT	Heart Disease

FOOD IDIOSYNCRASIES

Quite a large number of the minor ailments that afflict us from day to day may very well be caused by the different food items we eat daily, through the mechanism called allergy. The different foods and their possible allergic reactions include the following:

	FOOD	POSSIBLE ALLERGY
1	Eggs	Eczema, GIT upset, migraine, anaphylaxis
2	Cow's milk	Urticaria, GIT upset, migraine, anaphylaxis
3	Fish	Urticaria, asthma, anaphylaxis
4	Soya beans	GIT upset, diarrhea (in children)
5	Tomatoes	Migraine
6	Oranges	Migraine
7	Banana	Migraine
8	Wheat	Migraine, eczema

To find out whether a particular ailment is due to food allergy or not, one should abstain from all foods (fast) for a few days and resume eating by introducing the different suspected items one at a time thereby monitoring which symptoms recur with which food item (the so-called "elimination diet").

It is important to bear in mind that food can be responsible for chronic diarrhoea in children.

FOOD SENSITIVITY AND FOOD ROTATION

When a particular food item is eaten regularly and over a long time, there is a tendency for the consumer to develop sensitivity to the particular food item. To avoid this, it is recommended that food rotation be practiced to avoid sensitivity and allergy.

SALT AND HEALTH

There are two types of salt: refined table salt and unrefined salt. Refined salt is the salt sold in the market, while sea salt is sold as deep sea salt.

Refined salt is toxic to the body and triggers many degenerative diseases including hypertension, diabetes, stroke, arthritis, glaucoma, cancer, kidney failure and heart disease.

On the other hand, unrefined sea salt must be made an inseparable part of a healthy diet. The benefits of sea salt include:

e.   Carries nutrients to cells.

f.   Regulates blood pressure and volume.

g.   Facilitates digestion of food and absorption of nutrients.

h.   Keeps the body in harmony and balance.

The difference between refined table salt and sea salt is their tonic composition. While refined table salt contains 99% sodium chloride with 1% iodine, unrefined salt contains 100% macro trace elements such as; 84% sodium chloride, 14% magnesium, calcium and potassium and the remaining 2% is made up of other essential elements.

While refined table salt causes elevation of blood pressure, unrefined sea salt lowers high blood pressure and normalizes over time. It restores good digestive allergies and skin diseases. It restores good digestion especially in the elderly. Unrefined salt also eliminates excess sodium form the body and prevents fluid accumulation.

Other benefits of unrefined salt are: prevents the body against chronic illness, mild chronic dehydration, normalizes hormonal balance in the body and controls hypertension, diabetes mellitus and muscle strength.

CHAPTER 21
WHAT ABOUT MONOSODIUM GLUTAMATE (MSG)?

Monosodium glutamate or MSG as it is popularly known is the major constituent of virtually all "modern" seasonings.

Monosodium glutamate is made up of chemical portions: sodium and glutamate. The sodium part exerts the same effect on the human body as sodium chloride or table salt. In other words, regular excessive use of MSG can predispose some people to developing high blood pressure.

It can also worsen hypertension in those who already have the disease. And for those who have diseases of the heart or liver where table salt is restricted, MSG is automatically contraindicated, as it can also cause exacerbation of these medical conditions.

The glutamate portion of MSG is an amino acid which is thought to be the cause of drowsiness, headache, dizziness and other unpleasant feelings –the so-called ''Chinese Restaurant Syndrome'' seen in some people after excessive use of MSG. Although these reactions to MSG last from a few minutes to a few hours, they can recur with each meal containing MSG, and this is often mistaken for more serious disease. For the clinicians therefore, a symptom that is absent in the morning but build up later in the day and reach a crescendo in the afternoon, food allergy or sensitivity (especially to MSG) must be excluded as plausible cause.

Moreover, the glutamate, acting like adrenaline, releases sugar from the stores in the liver and makes glucose unavailable when it is needed later. This is thought to be the underlying cause of chronic, intractable body weakness and lethargy like chronic fatigue syndrome (CFS) in some people who use MSG.

MSG has also been shown to cause adult or late onset asthma in susceptible individuals. So that for any patient presenting with adult onset asthma, therefore clinicians should exclude MSG as a possible cause.

In summary therefore, MSG is a most unhealthy food item that should be avoided as much as possible for health and life-long vitality. Formy patients who complain of chronic lethargy, intractable body weakness, headaches, dizziness and other unpleasant feelings in the body, I usually ask them to avoid MSG for a week; if the condition does not improve, then I set about investigating them for more serious illness.

Very recently in India, a research finding discovered that MSG cubes were loaded with the heavy toxic metal –lead. This is an urgent call for NAFDAC to step in and investigate the common seasoning cubes in markets across the country.

A healthier and better seasoning item for regular use in all homes is the local locust beans seed, which is common to most communities in Nigeria. In northern Nigeria, it is called dadawa and the Yoruba's call it iru. Its salt content is very low but it is rich in potassium and calcium. In fact the high calcium content of dadawa is thought to be one contributory factor to the low incidence of osteoporosis in African women who eat meals seasoned with this traditional seasoning.

CHAPTER 22
ANTI-INFLAMMATORY FOODS

"He who takes medicine and neglects to diet wastes the skill of his doctors"
(Chinese Proverb)

Current scientific thinking agrees that inflammation is a common aetiology of many chronic diseases, with oxidative stress as the antecedent that fans the inflammatory response. The inflammation is thought to underlie diseases such as rheumatoid arthritis, valvular heart disease, chronic degenerative diseases, immune disease, diabetes, systemic lupus, erythematosis, multiple sclerosis, inflammatiory bowel disease, asthma, coronary artery disease, arteriosclerosis, Alzheimer's disease, and Parkinson's disease. Recently, scientists are beginning to also link cancer with abnormal inflammatory response to oxidative stress.

This new hypothesis for age-related disease has opened up a new and simple way of modifying or preventing this large group of diseases that form the main barrier to health, aging and longevity. This has also led to the newest subspecialty of "anti-aging medicine" that is rapidly helping this segment of aging population to live longer and healthier lives as opposed to geriatrics which, like most orthodox medical specialties, wait for people to get sick before loading them with drugs.

The inflammatory process is under the control of pituitary hormones and as long as the hormones are working optimally, the risk of chronic inflammatory diseases, including cancer, is significantly reduced.

This is why some people are postulating that if one can stimulate the pituitary gland appropriately with the right foods, to keep producing hormones optimally through correct feeding, the life expectancy of man can be extended indefinitely. This may be an overstatement but it underpins the fundamental importance of eating the correct foods that will stimulate the pituitary gland with foods that are naturally anti-inflammatory in nature – the so-called anti-inflammatory foods. The nutrients that are directly concerned with inflammatory response in the body are fats and phytonutrients.

a.   Fats: fats that are pre-inflammatory and disease prone include those that are rich in omega 6 fatty acid. They include:

1.   Chicken fat – agric. chicken (grain-fed)
2.   Most commercial vegetable oils in the market
3.   Grain-fed animals (agricultural animals)

Fats that oppose inflammation i.e. anti-inflammatory oils are those that are rich in omega – 3 fatty acid. They are hard to come by and include:

a.   Leaf green (small)
b.   Walnut
c.   Flaxseed
d.   Hemp
e.   Soyabean oil
f.   Canola oil
g.   Sea vegetables
h.   Fish (salmon, sardines, herring mackerel)
i.   Grass-fed animals (bushmeat not smoked)

To enjoy good health devoid of chronic inflammatory diseases, the ratio of omega-3 to omega-6 in the diet should be almost 1:1 or better 2:1 in favour of omega -3 in order to prevent most chronic illnesses, including cancer.

The typical western diet (and urban diet in Nigeria) has the ratio of omega -3 to omega -6 to be 1:20 in favor of omega-6. This explains the very high prevalence of chronic non-communicable diseases where over 75% of the populations are grappling with one chronic disease or the other. The problem is particularly grievous in the elderly where most of the last twenty or so years of their so called prolonged life expectancy is burdened by one form of disease or the other. The main sources of the omega-6 include:

1.   Fast foods
2.   Grain-fed cows
3.   High red meat diet relative to fish
4.   Junk foods like bread, biscuits, crackers, cookies, cakes, candy

Omega-6 loaded foods listed above predispose to diseases such as asthma, coronary artery disease, many forms of cancer, autoimmune disease and neurodegenerative disease.

In addition to omega-3 to omega-6 ratio, some foods are inherently evil nutritionally, directly causing disease when eaten regularly. They include:

a.   Margarine
b.   Partially hydrogenated vegetable oil (trans-fats)
c.   Vegetable shortening (vegetable fat)

Simple rules to avoid bad fats (and chronic diseases):

1. Read food labels: avoid any food labeled partially hydrogenated oil as an ingredient
2. Do not use vegetable shortenings
3. Never eat margarine
4. Avoid fried foods
5. Avoid any oil or food that smells rancid
6. Eat very little soya bean oil or any polyunsaturated oil for that matter (safflowers, sunflowers , corn, sesame)
7. Never heat oil to the point of smoking
8. Never reuse oil that has been heated to high temperatures

Most vegetable oils in our supermarkets are extracted with high temperatures and using hydrocarbon solvents that create pro-inflammatory products

The only oils recommended for regular consumption include extra virgin olive oil, avocado oil, atili oil, natural butter (Fulani) oil.

To separate caffeine from polyphenols in green tea

1. Steep 2 bags in hot water for thirty seconds, change the water and throw it away. This removes most caffeine.
2. Then put fresh hot water in the cup and steep the 2 tea bags for 2 – 3 minutes only and drink all of it. Always buy organic varieties of your green tea from the internet or from known manufacturers.

Other anti-inflammatory foods to eat for healthy disease-free living

1. Ginger
2. Turmeric
3. Cabbage
4. Broccoli

Arginine and Health

Arginine stimulates the pituitary gland to produce hormones that maintain youthfulness for life. It constitutes 80% of male seminal fluid.

Foods that are rich in arginine include:

1. Peanuts (not good for blood group O)
2. Cashew nuts
3. Watermelon seeds

4.	Walnuts
5.	Green leaves (celery)
6.	Garlic
7.	 Ginseng
8.	Red wine
9.	Root Vegetables (yam, sweet potatoes)

Histidine

It is particularly useful for sexual arousal in women. Common local sources include: banana, grapes, yams, sweet potatoes and green leaves.

Cooked Foods and Health

Cooked foods are deranged, denatured and destroyed to the extent they are cooked. Cooking destroys vitamins, enzymes and deaminates amino acids. It reduces minerals to unsuitable inorganic states, camaralises sugars and renders fats to become carcinogenic, pyrrolated hydrocarbons and acroleins.

CHAPTER 23
PLANNING THE SUPER-NUTRITION DIET

"We command nature only by obeying her"

(Bacon)

In previous chapters, I have tried to remind readers of the nutritional values of the common food items in the country and also explain the functions of each class of food and their constituent nutrients.

In this chapter, I shall go on to demonstrate how the knowledge of nutrition so acquired can be used to plan a diet that will confer health and vitality on all who care to adopt it.

To confer life-long vitality, a diet must be planned to achieve the following basic criteria:

- It must be nutritionally adequate in terms of carbohydrates (70% calories), vitamins (30g), minerals, fibre, proteins (10%) and fats (20%).
- It must be eaten at the right time, in the right quantity and quality.
- It should be palatable.

BREAKFAST

Based on the points raised in earlier chapters, the list of foods to be selected from for breakfast is as follows:

1.   CARBOHYDRATES

(a)   Yam

(b)   Plantain

(c)   Sweet potato (best eaten boiled in-skin)

(d)   Irish potato

(e)   Cocoyam

(f)   Wheat (home-baked bread)

(g)   Brown rice

(h)   Acha (gwate)

The above listed carbohydrates are best eaten boiled. The heat from boiling gives carbohydrates the same "pepping-up" effect equivalent to or even better than the effect of drinking a cup of tea or coffee in the morning.

2.   PROTEINS

(a)   Beans

(b)   Eggs

(c)   Fish

(d)   Red meat

(e)   Milk/yoghurt and cheese depending on blood group

3.   FATS

The amount of vegetable oil used to make sauce for eating with complex carbohydrates listed above is enough to supply all the fat requirements for the day. Remember, an average person requires only 3-6 teaspoonfuls of oil per day. Most commercial vegetable oils in the market are made from heating palm oil to very high degrees of temperature in factories. These heated or refined oils are particularly unhealthy because the heating destroys their vitamin E content, which is so important as an anti-oxidant in the body. Moreover, heating fats and oils renders them carcinogenic due to pyrrolated hydrocarbons and acrolein. This is one of the most important reasons why deep fried foods are so harmful and must be avoided for good health. Almost of all factory-processed vegetable oils contain potentially harmful chemicals and additives that preclude their regular consumption. The healthiest oils to use in order of preference are cold-pressed extra virgin coconut oil, avocado oil, olive oil, atili oil, flaxseed oil and little palm oil.

LUNCH

It is traditional in most Nigerian families to eat rice and beans at lunch and save the heavy meals like pounded yam, amala, eba, or tuwo for supper. This is nutritionally topsy-turvy and should be changed nationally. For good health, we need to change this attitude for an overall improvement of health. Heavy meals should be eaten in the morning and afternoons. Evening meals must be decidedly and deliberately, very light. The lighter, the healthier. The following foods are most suitable for eating at lunch.

1.   HEAVY MEAL(Starchy Carbohydrate)

(a)   Pounded yam

(b)   Tuwo (Acha, guinea corn)

(c)   Amala

(d)   Eba

(e)   Banana

(f)   Cocoyam

(g)   Sweet potato

(h)   Tuwo (brown rice)

(i)   Madidi

(j)   Alibo

2.   PROTEIN

(a)   Beans

(b)   Beef (small quantity)

(c)   Fish (ad libertim)

(d)   Egusi soup

(e)   Bushmeat

(f)   Fura da nono

3.   FATS

The amount of olive oil used to make soup is enough daily requirement of oil for most people. Remember to eat coconut oil and butter (Fulani) very sparingly only, but they should not be avoided completely.

4.   FRUITS AND VEGETABLES

Popular Nigerian vegetable soups like edikaikon, baobab leaves, beniseed leaves, okro leaves, and bitter leaves are all excellent food items that should be eaten daily, if possible. For instance, as stated earlier, baobab leaf (miyan kuka) is very rich in fibre, calcium, iron and phosphorus. It is also an excellent food for growing children, pregnant women and lactating mothers.

DINNER

For all-round vitality, no one should eat after 7.30pm. Supper time should range between 6.30pm and 7.30pm. The food should be very light always. If there's any desire for more food after the evening meal, this should be in the form of fruits and vegetables only.

1.   Carbohydrates:

(a)   Brown Rice (jollof, boiled or white but never fried)

2.   Protein

(a)   Fish (eat as fresh fish pepper soup not fried)

(b)   Chicken (as boiled pepper soup not fried)

(c)   Soybean soup

(d)   Beans (boiled or moi moi)

(e)   Seafoods (once in a while only)

3.   **FRUITS AND VEGETABLES**: These form the hub of the life-long vitality diet. It actually revolves around fruits and vegetables. This is true because recent scientific findings show that they supply the longevity substance, fibre. They also contain nutrients, especially vitamins. Vegetables also contain anti-cancer factors that protect the body against cancerous growths.

In view of their huge importance, therefore, fruits and vegetables constitute the honorable permanent representatives at every meal. They can be eaten as much as one desires without serious ill-effects. The only source of concern about too much vegetables is that they tend to prevent the absorption of certain important minerals due to their phytate content.

To overcome this important dilemma, therefore, it is advised that one limits the quantity of vegetables to a particular meal in a day. For instance, one may decide to have fruits alone without vegetables at breakfast, and eat vegetables at lunch. Otherwise, the diet should be as mixed as possible to reduce the problem of phytates to a minimum. The following is the list of common available fruits and vegetables to choose from for daily consumption in order to ensure life-long vitality:

1.   Oranges
2.   Water-melon
3.   Pawpaw
4.   Grape fruit
5.   Guava
6.   Cucumber
7.   Green beans
8.   Apples
9.   Mangoes
10.   Tomatoes
11.   Pineapple
12.   Onions
13.   Garlic
14.   Lemon
15.   Lime
16.   Lettuce
17.   Cabbage
18.   Carrots

19. Pepper
20. Spinach
21. Pumpkin

The actual amount of vegetables and fruits in the traditional African diet ranges from 60 – 160g/day only; this is very poor indeed. This is because the WHO stipulates that for good health, a person needs to consume at least 400g of fruits and vegetables per day. It is speculated that this paucity might be the explanation for the very short life-expectancy of Africans (47 years as compared to 84 years in Japan). To improve our life expectancy at birth, therefore, the government should encourage farmers in the cultivation of fruits and vegetables and encourage the people to eat them more liberally.

New way to live longer

Eating sparingly: Eating ¼ of what you eat currently will make you live healthier and longer. Cutting your calorie intake by just ¼ will reduce your chances of getting cancer, lower your fasting blood sugar, lower your resting body temperature as well as your resting heart rate. The general outcome is a very vibrant and zestful life into ripe old age.

To cut down your total calorie intake, a person must avoid high calorie foods like processed flour foods (amala, eba, alibo and powdered cereals) which are generally 300 calories per 100g or above. One should rather concentrate on fresh starchy root carbohydrate (70%) like pounded yam, boiled sweet potatoes, cocoyam and yam. These have low food energy concentration ranging from 110 to 150 calorie per 100g.

CHAPTER 24
JUSTIFICATION FOR THE SUPER-NUTRITION DIET

"The discovery of a healthful dish is more important to humanity than the discovery of a distant galaxy"

(Salmette Guerin)

I have spent the last 30 years trying to perfect a superior diet that will provide all the essential 91 nutrients as at when needed by the body in order to live disease-free and timeless. The meals are first and foremost blood group-compatible. They are also well timed and the different foods to be eaten in particular order in the right quantity and quality.

The meals are scientifically planned to be adequate in terms of energy content (70% starchy carbohydrate, 10% protein and 20% fats/oils). The total fibre content of the meal in 24 hours is 35g or more as recommended for the prevention of diseases like cancer, obesity, diabetes, and arthritis. The vitamin and mineral content of the meals meet their recommended daily allowance. Finally, the life-long vitality diet is based on commonly available natural foods so that a person does not need to bore a hole in his or her pocket to eat them regularly.

The following tables (1-3) and their analyses will further clarify and demonstrate the super level and beauty of the diet.

THOMAS AFFI BREAKFAST SALAD (TABS)

S/N	ACRONYM	FOOD ITEM	PORTION (g)	PORTION SIZE	QUANTITY	ENERGY (CALORIES)	CARBOHYDRATE (g)	PROTEIN (g)	FATS (g)	FIBRES (g)
1	G	Green leaves (Spinach)	90	½ cooked	1 cup	21	3	3	0	2
2	L	Lemon juice	54	Raw	½ lemon	17	5	1	0	2
3	O	Olive oil	13.5	Raw	1 tbspn	119	0	0	14	0
4	B	Beetroot	170	Raw	1 cup	65	15	2	t	1
5	B	Banana	456	Raw	2 fingers	242	54	2	2	6
6	A	Apple cider vinegar	15	Raw	1 tbspn	0	1	0	0	0
7	C	Carrot	72	½ cooked	1 meduim	30	4	0	0	3
8	C	Cabbage	145	½ cooked	1 cup	30	6	2	t	4
9	A	Avocado	50.25	Raw	1	81	3.75	1	8.25	4

10	S	Sunflower seeds	10	Raw	10g	57	1.88	2.29	4.9	1.1
11	E	Egg	50	Hard-boiled	1	78	1	6	5	0
12	B	Beans	340	Cooked	1 cup	217	40	12	1	12.2
	U									
13	S	Sesame (black)	10	Raw	10g	57	2.36	1.8	5	1.5
14	T	Tomato	123	Raw	1 (medium)	26	6	1	0	1
15	O	Onions	79.9	Raw	1 (medium)	30	7	1	0	1
16	S	Sweet pepper (red or green)	74	Raw	1 (medium)	20	5	1	t	1.2
17	S	Starch (sweet potato)	462	Cooked	3 (medium)	510	120	9	3	9.9
SUB-TOTAL						1668.67	275.0	45.1	43.2	69.0
TOTAL				82% Raw		-	65.9%	10.8%	23.3%	-

THOMAS AFFI MIRACLE SHAKE (TAMS)

S/N	FOOD ITEM	RAW OR COOKED	PORTION SIZE	TOTAL FIBRE (g)	ENERGY (CALORIES)	CARBOHYD RATE(g)	PROTEIN(g)	FATS(g)
1	Bitterleaf	Raw	1 cup	5.8		29	18.4	1.6
2	Brewer's yeast	Raw	1 tbspn	2.2	25	3	3	0
3	Carrot	Raw	1 stick	3	50	11	1	T
4	Cabbage	Raw	1 cup	4	30	6	1	t
5	Lemon juice	Raw	½ lemon	0.3	30	10.5	0.5	t
6	Brown sugar	Cooked	1 tablespoon	0	52	13	0	0
7	Moringa leaves	Raw	1 cup	0.9	92	12.5	6.7	1.7
8	Turmeric	Raw	½ teaspoon	0.1	11	2.1	0.2	0.2
9	Wheatgerm oil	Raw	1 tbspn	0	119	0	0	14
10	Broccoli	Raw	1 cup	2.5	35	6	4	t
11	Cauliflower	Raw	1 cup	2.4	27	5	2	t
12	Cucumber	Raw	1 (medium)	2.5	27	3	1	t
13	Celery	Raw	1 cup	2.4	22	5	1	t
14	Parsley	Raw	½ cup	0.2	1	t	t	t

15	Radish	Raw	½ cup	0.1	5	t	t	t
16	Pomegranate juice	Raw	30 ml	1.1	105	t	t	1
	TOTAL	**95% Raw**						

Choose first 10 and add any four from the rest based on blood group compatibility and availability.

LUNCH TABLE

S/NO	ACRONYM	FOOD ITEM	RAW OR COOKED	PORTION SIZE	TOTAL FIBRE (g)	ENERGY (CALORIES)	CARBOHYDRATE (g)	PROTEIN(g)	FATS(g)
FRUITS AND SALAD									
1		Fruits (water melon)	Raw	1 cup	0.7	74	16.9	0.6	0.4
2	S	Spinach	½ cooked	1 cup	2	21	3	3	0
3	L	Lettuce	Raw	1 cup	0	9	1	1	1
4	O	Onions	Raw	1 medium	1	30	1	1	0
5	T	Tomato	Raw	1 medium	1	26	1	1	0
6	R	Radish	Raw	4 medium	1	5	t	t	t
7	A	Asparagu	Raw	½ cup	0	15	2	2	0
8	C	Cabbage	Raw	1 cup	0	17	1	1	0
9	C	Cucumber	Raw	7 slices	1	5	0	0	0
10	C	Celery	Raw	1 stalk	1	5	t	t	t
MAIN DISH									
11		Boiled yam	Cooked	2 handful	3.3	158	38	2	t
12		Pounded yam	Cooked	Fist	0.6	98.4	23	1.5	t
13		Guinea corn	Cooked	Fist	1.8	405.5	84	11.3	2.7
14		Brown rice	Cooked	Fist	3.3	227	45	5	2
15		Millet	Cooked	Fist	2.0	312	78	9.1	4.6
16		Hungry rice (Acha)	Cooked	Fist	0.4	392	88	7.14	1.3
17		Soup (Egusi, Okra)	Cooked	1 cup	2	51	12	3	t
18		Lean Beef	Cooked	100g	0	130	0	19.1	8.1
19		Chicken Breast	Cooked	100g	0	150	0	20	6.4
20		Fish	Cooked	100g	0	50	2	5	3
SPICES AND CONDIMENTS									
21	G	Garlic	Raw						
22	B	Basil	Raw						
23	O	Oregano	Raw						
24	M	Marjoram	Raw						

S/N	Acronym	Food Item	Raw or Cooked	Portion Size	Total Fibre(g)	Calories Total(g)	Carbohydrate(g)	Protein(g)	Fats(g)
25	P	Parsley	Raw						
26	L	Lemon juice	Raw						
27	A	Apple cider vinegar	Raw						
28	S	Sea salt	Raw						
29	T	Thyme	Raw						
		TOTAL	**70% Raw**						

DINNER/SUPPER TABLE

S/N	ACRONYM	FOOD ITEM	RAW OR COOKED	PORTION SIZE	TOTAL FIBRE(g)	CALORIES TOTAL(g)	CARBOHYDRATE(g)	PROTEIN(g)	FATS(g)
SALAD									
1	S	Spinach	½ cooked	1 cup	2	21	3	3	0
2	L	Lettuce	Raw	1 cup	0	9	1	1	1
3	O	Onions	Raw	1 medium	1	30	1	1	0
4	T	Tomato	Raw	1 medium	1	26	1	1	0
5	R	Radish	Raw	4 medium	1	5	T	t	t
6	A	Asparagu	Raw	½ cup	0	15	2	2	0
7	C	Cabbage	Raw	1 cup	0	17	1	1	0
8	C	Cucumber	Raw	7 slices	1	5	0	0	0
9	C	Celery	Raw	1 stalk	1	5	T	t	t
MAIN DISH									
10		Brown rice	Cooked	2 handful	3.3	216	225	20	18
11		Quaker oats	Cooked	2 cups	24.6	130	23	5	2
12		Fruits (in season)	Raw	2 cups	1.2	102	24	2	2
13		Honey	Raw	1 teaspoon	-	65	17	t	0
14		Red wine/Juice	Cooked	1 glass	0	21	1	t	0
15		Olive oil	Cooked	1 tbspn	0	120	0	0	14
16		Apple (½ red)	Cooked	½ apple	1.2	40	15	t	t
17		Yoghurt	Raw	100g	0	615	45	4.8	4.5
18		Fura	-	110g	0.39	-	29.4	6.25	2.14
19		Tea (Chamomile, Sage, Dandelion)	-	1 cup					
SPICES AND CONDIMENTS									
20	G	Garlic	Raw						
21	G	Basil	Raw						
22	O	Oregano	Raw						
23	M	Marjoram	Raw						

24	P	Parsley	Raw						
25	L	Lemon juice	Raw						
26	A	Apple cider vinegar	Raw						
27	S	Sea salt	Raw						
28	T	Thyme	Raw						
		TOTAL	**80% Raw**						

ANALYSIS OF THOMAS AFFI LONGEVITY DIET

The Thomas Affi Longevity Diet (TAL Diet) above (TABS, TAMS, LUNCH and DINNER) is a beautiful summary of the arguments and persuasions put forward in this book in favour of a simple, practical diet that is versatile and meets all the attributes of an optimum diet in terms of its taste, nutrient complement, protein, fat, energy distribution throughout the day as well as its fibre content being hither to the most difficult and elusive good dietary component to achieve. TAL Diet also represents my earnest and humble attempt to come up with a diet or programme that is unique and distinct in its providing over 70% of total food consumed raw, unprocessed, fresh and locally available. The aim is to meet the daily human requirements for 91 nutrients as well as to address squarely the perennial flaws of existing diets that have courted much ill-health, leading to poor health indices, high morbidity and avoidable premature deaths. The diet by design addresses the blood and its circulation, the heart and cardiovascular system. When the heart and cardiovascular system are intact and functioning optimally, the rest of the body will follow suit.

TOTAL CALORIE SUMMARY OF THOMAS AFFI LONGEVITY DIET

S/N		MEAL	CARBOHYDRATE	PROTEIN	FAT	FIBRE	ENERGY (Calorie)	% ENERGY
1		**TABS**	275.0g	45.1g	43.2g	69.0g	1668.67	56
2		**TAMS**	62.0g	14.0g	16.0g	13.4g	448.0	15.1
3		**LUNCH**	58.9g	15.1g	3.4g	8.3g	326.6	11

4	**DINNER**	95.0g	14.8g	8.5g	5.7g	515.7	17
	TOTAL (grams)	490.89g	89.0g	71.1g	96.4g	2959.0	-
	SUB-TOTAL (CALORIES)	1963.56	356.0	639.9	-	2959.0	-
	%TOTAL CALORIES/DAY	66.4	12.03	21.6	-	-	100

It is recommended that for good health and longevity, a person should eat foods of different colours, the so-called "rainbow diet". The very wide variety of food colours in the TAL diet has put it in a class of its own, being nutritionally accurate and scientifically up-to-date.

Finally, nutrition experts further recommend that for a diet to be adequate and wholesome, it should capture within it, the six common tastes: sour, bitter, sweet, pungent, salty and astringent. Heartily again, the TAL diet has all the six tastes represented.

To further applaud the beauty of the diet, I wish to present as follows;

A. **Breakfast:** For good health, nutritional scientists agree across board that a person should eat breakfast like a king, lunch like a prince and dinner like a pauper. In other words, the biggest and richest meal of the day should be breakfast; lunch should be moderate and dinner very light. The T.A.L Diet by design meets the above aspirations most faithfully; with the breakfast providing 66.4%, lunch 26% and dinner 17% of total calories consumed in a day.

B. **Total Energy for 24 Hours:** the TAL Diet again has scored excellently in terms of total energy provision over 24 hours that turned out to be 2,959 calories, being very close to the average energy requirement of an active woman (2,500) and an active man (3,500). For persons who are concerned about their weight or simply want to restrict calorie intake, the lunch can be either TAMS alone or the main Lunch alone and not both. This will go a long way to reduce the total calorie intake without compromising the diet.

C. **Protein Content:** Edward Smith, a British physician who studied energy and protein metabolism in 1862 concluded that a physically active man needs 80g of protein daily. During the next 40 years, other estimates of protein needs ranged up to a maximum of 150g per day with a lower limit of 35g/day. The current best estimate for protein need is 0.8g/day per body weight (kg). This works out to be 56g/day for a man of 70kg and 44g/day for an average woman of 55kg. This RDA of protein intake is too high for diabetics and persons with renal insufficiency. On the other hand, if elderly people eat too little protein, they tend to suffer marked loss of muscle mass; making them look much older than their chronological age. But the increase in protein intake of elders should be mainly of plant origin (legumes) and not animal protein because animal protein increases calcium loss in urine leading to osteoporosis and its serious consequences. Edward Smith's estimate above comes close to TAL diet recommendation of 89.0g/day which applies particularly in pregnant women, growing children and the elderly.

The protein content of the TAL Diet is therefore, another very big plus for the protocol. First and foremost, the protein is largely of plant origin, making it virtually free from saturated fat and cholesterol. Secondly, the total protein energy is only 12% of the total calorie consumed in 24 hours, making the diet kidney and liver friendly, enabling these important organs to perform optimally without depreciation into ripe old age. The last but not the least important aspect of the protein component is that it provides 89g of protein per 24 hours which makes it ideal to support the immunity of elderly person to resist infection for years on end.

D. **Fats and Oils:** Here again, the TAL Diet has demonstrated very clearly that it is a super nutrition dynamo with the fat content being beautifully within the scientifically recommended range of 20g-25g/day for healthy adults without cardiovascular risks. The 21% total fat calorie content of the diet is also ideal. Moreover, almost 80% of the fat is of plant origin, with little or no cholesterol or saturated fats. This is another very big plus indeed for the diet.

E. **Starch/Grain Carbohydrate:** Bread used to be known as the 'staff of life', butcurrent nutritional opinion stronglyis of the view that it is unprocessed starch and grains that are truly the 'staff of life' and not bread which is a highly processed complex carbohydrate. It is now believed that unprocessed starch and whole grain carbohydrates can prevent and/ or even cure most of the common modern diseases like diabetes, obesity, hypertension, atherosclerosis, stroke, heart and kidney diseases.

Far from being villains therefore, unprocessed starchy roots and whole grains foods are nutritional angels that should constitute at least 70% of our daily fare as obtained in rural African communities (see table below).

LIFE ON THOMAS AFFI LONGEVITY DIET

S/N	VARIABLE	U.K LIFE PROFILE		LIFE ON THOMAS AFFI DIET
		1900	1990	
1	Life expectancy (years)	48 years	71 years	128 years (projected)
2	Work week (days)	6 days	5 days	5 days
3	Food income/allocation	46%	20%	30%
4	Protein intake (g/day)	71g	69g	89g (80% plant)
5	Carbohydrate intake(g/day)	375g	246g	490.89g (90% unprocessed starch and grains)
6	Fats intake(g/day)	65g	98g	71g (80% plant)
7	Fibre intake(g/day)	20g	15g	96.4g (prevents/ cures modern disease)
8	Time to run 100 yards	22sec	9.8sec	9.0sec (projected)

F. **Fibre:** Most gratifying is the fact that the diet is decidedly rich in fibre (96.4g/day), which is the glorious distinction about the recommended diet. I have not known of any diet that has achieved this degree of nutritional splendor. Low fibre diet of most developed societies has been associated with obesity, heart disease, artheresclerosis, hypertension, colorectal cancer, diverticulosis of the gut and many others. On the other hand, the high fibre diets of the rural community of the developing world are associated with near absence of all the diseases listed for low fibre diet. For instance in 1960s, missionary doctors working in Kampala, Uganda, Dr. Denis Burkitt and Dr. H.C Trommell noticed the Africans were remarkably free from high blood pressure, heart disease, diabetes, obesity and other western disorders including constipation, appendicitis, diverticulosis, heamorrhoids, hernias and gallstones. The doctors had also observed that their African patients had much more rapid and bulky bowel movements than their British counterparts. These simple observations led to the theory that high fibre (150g/day for Uganda and 130g/day for Kenya) protect against many of the intestinal, metabolic and cardiovascular disorders that plague industrialized societies.

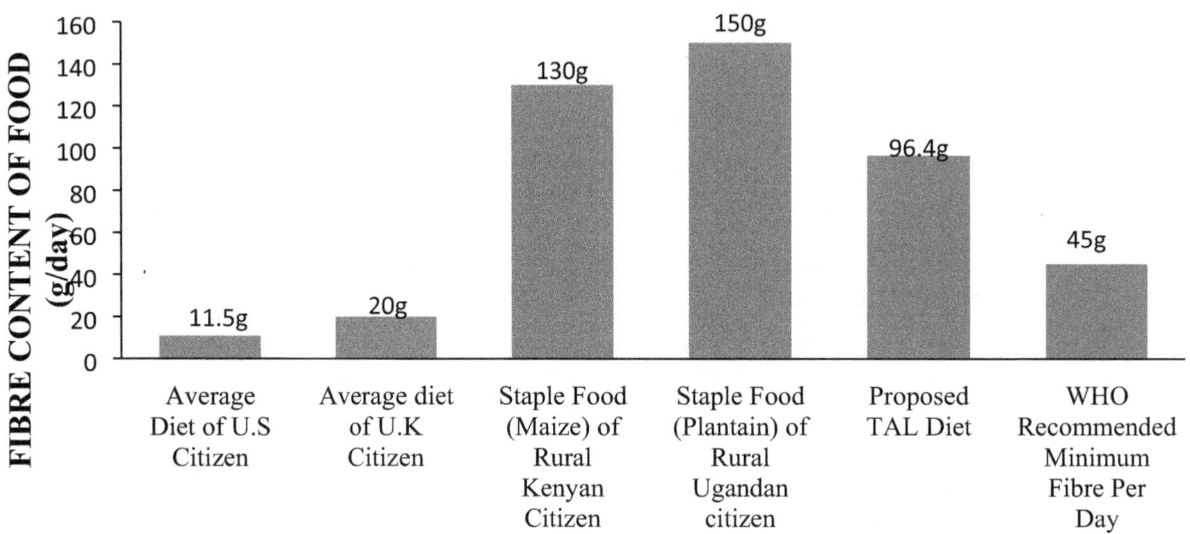

A Chart Showing the Fibre Contents of Average Diets of Developed and Developing Communities Compared with the Minimum of WHO and the Ideal of Thomas Affi Longevity Diet.

HEALING PROPERTIES OF SOME COMMON FOODS

S/N	ACTIVITY	FOOD SOURCES	REMARKS
1	Anti-aging	Spinach, Carrot, Pawpaw, Sweet Pepper (Green or White)	Fully provided for in our diet tables
2	Anti-Alzheimers'	Dandelion, Peas, Soyabeans, Sunflower seeds, Lentils	Available in longevity diet
3	Anti-anxiety	Tomato, Broccoli, Valerian	Available in our longevity diet
4	Antiarrythmic	Cowpea, Lettuce, Oats, Radish, Spinach, Cucumber	All available in our longevity diet
5	Antiarthritic	Avocado, Cucumber, Sunflower, Evening Primrose, Sesame	Available in our longevity diet
6	Antiatherosclerotic	Evening Primrose, Broccoli, Tomato, Groundnut, Cabbage, Spinach	Available in our longevity diet
7	Antibackache	Cowpea, Balck Cohosh,	Available in our

		Asparagus, Spirulina, Sunflower Seeds, Black beans, Okra	longevity diet
8	Anticancer	Lemon, Celery, Orange, Lime, Thyme, Tomato, Sage, Cucumber, Broccoli, Carrot, Parsley	All fully available in our diet
9	Anticarcinogenic	Mango, Asparagus, Green Peas, Pomegranate	Fully provided for in our protocol
10	Anticariogenic	Grapes, Lemon, Thyme, Coriander, Green Tea	Fully represented in our diet
11	Anticataract	Evening Primrose, Sunflower Seeds, Bitter Melon, Strawberry	Fully represented in diet
12	Anticirrhotic	Milk Thistle, Turmeric, Cordyceps, Vitamin E, Fenugreek, Soyabeans, Dandelion	Fully provided for in the proposed diet
13	Antidepressant	Asparagus, Lettuce, Spinach, Cowpea, Tomato, Quaker Otas	All available in diet
14	Antidiabetic	Thyme, Dandelion, Cinnamon, Dates	Available in diet
15	antifatigue	Lettuce, Asparagus, Ginseng, Cowpea, Radish, Cabbage, Oats, Spinach, Dandelion, Cucumber	Fully provided for in the proposed diet
16	Antiglaucoma	Celery, Parsley, Bitter Melon	Available in proposed diet
17	Antihypertensive	Evening Primrose, Lettuce, Asparagus, Cowpea, Radish, Cabbage, Oats, Dill, Dandelion, Spinach	Available in proposed diet
18	Antihyperthyroid	Thyme, Blackbeans, Lettuce, Orange, Grapefruits, Cabbage, Asparagus, Spinach, Parsley	All commonly available and provided for in the longevity diet
19	Anti-impotency	Lettuce, Spinach, Parsley, Oats, Brown Rice, Millet	Fully provided for in the longevity diet

20	Anti-lupus	Cabbage, Spinach, Carrot	Fully covered in diet
21	Antimelanomic	Grapes, Lemon, Thyme, Asparagus, Green Pea, Oregano	Fairly covered in diet
22	Antiosteo-arthritis	Bell Pepper, Cayenne Pepper, Horseradish, Cashew, English Walnuts, Guava	Fairly covered in diet
23	Antioxidants	Pawpaw, Dates, Pomegranate, Carrot, Water	Available and covered in diet
24	Antiparkinsonian	Broad Bean, Sunflower Seeds, Asparagus, Spinach, Soyabeans, Peas, Cabbage	Available and fully covered in diet
25	Antirheumatic	Sunflower Seeds, Lemon, Thyme, Evening Primrose, Asparagus, Pea	Available and covered in diet
26	Antischizophrenic	Fenugreek, Avocado, Peas, American Ginseng, Sweet Potato, Brown Rice, Sesame, Soyabeans	Available and covered in diet
27	Antistress	Parsnips, Parsley, Fenugreek, Ginseng, Carrot	Fairly covered in diet
28	Antitumor	Lemon, Thyme, Celery, Evening Primrose, Dates	Available and covered in diet
29	Cancer-preventive	Avocado, Celery, Thyme, Lemon In Green Tea, English Walnuts, Watermelon, Evening Primrose, Cucumber	Available and covered in diet
30	Cardiotonic	Green Tea, Guarana, Cayenne Pepper In Green Tea	Available and covered in diet
31	Hypoglycaemic	Green Tea, Evening Primrose, Ginseng, Garlic, Cinnamon, Onion, Periwinkle	Available and covered in diet
32	Hypotensive	Thyme, Evening Primrose, Dates, Moringa	Available and covered in diet
33	Immunostimulant	Dandelion, Sugar Beet	Available and covered in diet

The table above is just a sample. It is most gratifying to note from the remarks that the proposed longevity diet is fully versatile and practical which virtually prevents or treats various kinds of disease condition, making it an all-round health, dynamic and longevity.

In other words, by adhering to the proposed diet suggested in this chapter, one is guaranteed to live a vibrant, happy life without the fear of contracting the listed disease conditions and many more.

Take for instance cancer, it is often said that if one eats sparingly and sensibly, according to the proposed tables above, and at the same time, one adds antioxidant supplements to the diet, the chances of one developing cancer is almost zero.

CHAPTER 25
NON-FOOD HEALTHY PRACTICES

For all-round vivaciousness, correct nutrition must be complemented by certain non-food practices that are equally health promoting. They have been tried and tested and have been found to be extremely important for health upliftment and maintenance. These practices include: regular, moderate exercise, restful sleep at night, regular bowel opening and fasting for health.

REGULAR BOWEL OPENING

According to Herodius of Seylumbria, "a man whose bowels move regularly and normally will live long". This statement was made long ago before the Christian era but holds true to this day. Doctors and other health practitioners have long observed that health and vitality are closely related to a good appetite and regular bowel opening. The number of bowel openings per day is often in-born but can be regulated through proper diet, coupled with self-drilling over a few weeks.

The first and foremost requirement for regular bowel movement is the necessity for proper toning of the digestive tract through eating fibre-rich foods in the form of starchy carbohydrates, fresh fruits, vegetables, cereals, and legumes. Fibre is the singular most important factor responsible for day to day regular bowel opening.

The second most important factor in bowel opening is regular moderate exercise. Exercise tones up the gastro-intestinal muscles and makes regular bowel opening easy and fun.

The third and not the least important factor for regular bowel opening is adequate water drinking in the morning at least one hour before bowel opening – the so-called water therapy.

Regular bowel opening prevents prolonged contact of faeces with the bowel wall. Prolonged contact of faeces with the bowel wall causes irritation by toxic substances that are thought to cause cancer of the colon. The prolonged intestinal transit time also allows for absorption of toxins into the blood stream to cause ill-health. In view of the above two very important reasons, it is strongly advised that the bowels should be ideally opened three times a day to coincide with the three major daily propulsive actions of the gut that ensures movement of faeces from the rest of the intestine into the storage station in the left colon, sigmoid colon, and rectum. But because visiting the toilet three times a day is socially inconvenient for most people, opening of the bowel twice a day is near ideal. One should schedule the first bowel opening in the morning after breakfast because it is the entrance of food into the stomach that initiates propulsive action that empties the bowel; while the second bowel movement should be scheduled for evening after supper. Bowel movement is easier after a meal not before.

Most people, however, open their bowels once a day. This is acceptable too as long as the evacuation is total and completed in 3 phases – over 5 – 10 minutes. Bowel opening activity should be relaxed and pleasurable; never done hurriedly.

Adaptation to a new schedule of bowel movement may not come easily but one should not give up but keep on drilling oneself till one gets it right. At the initial stage one must suppress the urge to defecate at any other time other than the times selected. After a few weeks of drilling, the body soon adapts to the new health promoting schedule of two or more bowel openings in 24hours.

On the actual defecation process, one should never hurry the process. It should take at least 5–10 minutes (use the bathroom clock) for complete evacuation. At the initial stage, one may need to stay longer to get the stool out. But this should not discourage one from trying to acquire a regular bowel opening habit – one after breakfast and the other after dinner.

On the position for bowel opening, it is healthier to do it the African style-squatting-rather than the European style of sitting on a toilet seat. This is because, sitting is thought to encourage the development of hemorrhoids or piles, but squatting prevents pile development and allows for more complete bowel opening in view of the mechanical advantage inherent in the squatting position.

One very important point about regular bowel opening is that one can use it to serve as an early warning system to detect early onset of disease. This is especially true for diseases affecting the gastrointestinal tract. The reason being that bowel opening is one of the earliest things to change in disease situations. They become either too frequent or too few but seldom remain the same. This enables one to seek out medical help in good time whenever there's trouble. It was Henry Wheeler Shaw (1818 - 1885) who summarized the importance of bowel opening most succinctly as follows: "I have finally come to the conclusion that a good reliable set of bowels is worth more to a man than any quantity of brains".

FASTING

By fasting, I am not referring to the Christian lent period or the Muslim Ramadan fast. The fast I commend to you is not religious in its import per se, but is directly related to the life-long vitality programme advocated in this book. The fast here does not require any elaborate ceremonies or rituals.

The life-long vitality fast involves essentially the avoidance of solid foods and restricting one's meals to fruits and or plain water for the duration of the fast.

The one day fast usually begins at 6:00am and is broken at 6:00pm of the same day. Only fruits may be consumed at the usual meal-times. To make it less monotonous, it is advised that different varieties of fruits be consumed at the different times: breakfast, lunch and dinner. One is allowed to drink water during the fast: 300 ml every 3 hours. To avoid serious metabolic alkalosis which can complicate a diet of fruits taken alone for longer than two days, it is recommended that you restrict the fast to two or three consecutive days at a time (first three days of each month). It is also advisable to limit the fast to once a month.

For anyone who is not used to fasting, he or she is strongly advised to start with a half day fast, at least for the first month and increase to a full day the next month and to 24 hours subsequently. The half day fast begins at 6am and ends at 12:00 noon.

A good fast helps give the body the opportunity to clean out accumulated impurities that could otherwise clog the body systems and make them less efficient in the short term and cause disease in the long run.

Secondly, fasting is one of the surest ways of training one's self in the art of self-control and self-denial: the two traits that constitute the noblest pathway to health and vitality and nobility. On a more philosophical level, it is only through self-discipline that one can learn to control oneself. And once one can control oneself, one is automatically a master. And anyone who is a master of himself is by inference a master of the cosmos, since man is himself a microcosm of the cosmos. And no power under the sun can subdue a master of the cosmos except God, the creator.

Periodic fasts are wonderfully rejuvenating. Latest experiments with animals and men confirm extraordinary benefits of fasting in the cure of many ailments. The restoration of health and vitality, vigorous growth of hair, increased sexual power and general sense of well-being. As far back as the 18th century A.D. Thomas Tusser said it best: "Make hunger thy sauce, as medicine for health".

HEALING FAST

A stricter fast is often required for returning a diseased body back to normal by keeping away all poisons and allowing the inherent healing power of the body to take over. Such a healing fast requires abstinence from solid food 24 hours a day. Only small quantity of water–300ml–is allowed frequently every 3 hours throughout the fast.

According to H.L Anderson, such a fast can last up to six months under professional supervision in certain extreme cases of disease or for spiritual atonement. But ordinarily, fasts from 3 days to 4–5 weeks may be undertaken by experienced fasters without medical supervision. Beginners are, however, advised to stay within 3 – 7 days range. It is not true that one will die if one abstains from solid food 24 hours daily for a week or so.

To start such a strict fast, however, one does not just start off suddenly, but one is expected to train one's body to do with less and less food for 2 to 3 days before launching into total abstention.

One starts by gradually reducing food intake to juices and soups over a day or two. On the third, one eats nothing but only takes small amount of water frequently–one glass every hour.

During a fast, one is expected to carry on all normal activities including moderate exercises. The exercises should not be too heavy for the fasting person to tolerate.

To end a fast, one should reverse the starting protocol by taking fruit or vegetable juice on the first day of the 3 days to ending of the fast. Next day, light soup without any solids should be introduced. Small solid foods can be introduced on the third day and then normal food resumed as from the fourth day.

It is gratifying to observe that following a fast, the volume of the stomach significantly shrinks so that only small amount of food makes one feel satisfied. This may be beneficial to people who are over-weight and want to maintain their ideal body weight. This is far better than subjecting oneself to surgical reduction of the size of the stomach as done in some places for the treatment of obesity (bariatric surgery).

A healing fast on the other hand is touted to "cure" diseases; especially if water is taken in small quantities (100ml) every one hour throughout the fasting period.

REST

On the topic of rest for life-long vitality, I would like to quote Gordon MacDonald who said it most beautifully: "if my private world is in order, it must be because I have chosen to press Sabbath rest into the rush and routine of my daily life to find the rest God prescribed to himself and all humanity".

Most people are so busy making a living that they forget to live. Once in a while, it is vital to each one of us to take time off our striving and struggles and set aside a period during which one should just "lazy" around in bed doing absolutely nothing. The idea is to enable us rest physically, mentally and spiritually. The scriptures tell us God worked very hard six days to create the world but that on the seventh day, he rested. Not that God needed any rest as such, but he did it as a prescription for all humanity to observe for our health and vitality. The one day rest is expected to refresh the body, the soul and the spirit. It constitutes a rest-cure to enable us recuperate from the excesses of the week. During the one day Sabbath rest, one is expected to do absolutely nothing but rest for most of the day. One should restrict one's energy expenditure as much as possible including talking. One should eat light meals or even fast as I do on this rest-cure day – every Saturday (Sabbath).

A most convenient day for most people would be Saturday (Sabbath) since most people are absent from work on this day. Even though I am not a Seventh-day Adventist, I fast and rest from 6:00am to 6:00pm on Sabbath days. The next morning, I prepare and attend church service in honour of the resurrection of my Lord, Jesus Christ of Nazareth.

In addition to the once a week rest-cure day, it is vitally important to set aside 30 minutes to 1hr during work hours for complete rest from work during the day. This is needful for the body to rest from the standing or sitting position of work. One should lie flat, preferably on a bed, with the feet raised higher than the head. A sofa or long bench in the office would do very well. The ideal time for this rest is soon after eating lunch before one resumes work again. This should be nationally legislated to enable all workers rest for 1 hour after lunch as the French people do. The 1hour following lunch coincides with the sleepy moments that follow heavy meals. The sleepiness is physiologically due to the alkaline tide created in the body as a result of heavy acid secretion in the stomach necessary for digestion.

The position to adopt for the ½ hour rest is the prone or facedown position. Here, one should lie on one's stomach and chest face down: preferably tilted to one's left side so that one's heart is directly pressed down. This is the position that offers the least resistance to the work of the heart action and therefore the best position for the whole body to rest properly. When in this position of rest, one should practice deep breathing for at least 3 minutes at the beginning and at the end of the rest period. Deep breathing clears one's brain and revives one's spirit. Deep breathing also helps cure psychological tension and reduces high blood pressure. It is one of the mechanisms by which regular exercise lowers blood pressure and clears clinical depression and anxiety. Deep breathing is, indeed, the underlying healing principle attributed to yoga and other relaxation exercises for the cure of oxidative stress and psychosomatic diseases, especially the cure of the so-called executive stress.

EXERCISING FOR HEALTH

Regular physical exercise is the most crucial non-dietary pillar of the life-long vitality programme. Regular exercise encourages deep breathing that lowers peripheral resistance in blood vessels and thereby works to reduce blood pressure. One can eat all the fruits and vegetables, but if one is sedentary most of one's life, little can be gained in terms of health and vivaciousness. It is very important, especially for sedentary, white collar job workers, to engage in some form of physical exercise for 30 minutes at least three times a week. One can decide on any form of exercise that suits him or her but the exercise that cuts across age and gender is a brisk walk, lasting 20-30 minutes at least 3 -5 mornings or evenings a week.

In the tropics where the sun gets excessively hot most of the day, the best time for exercise is before sunrise and after sunset. I personally prefer early morning exercise for its convenience and for the very cool clean weather of the morning. The brisk walk should last 20-30 minutes a day and repeated every day or every other day. I have personally discovered that exercising every day can prove a bit exhausting, thereby defeating the very goals of the programme. I shall dwell more on this very important topic of exercising for life-long vitality in separate a book.

INTERMITTENT ANTIMICROBIALS AND LONGEVITY

Focal infections anywhere in the body can cause generalized ill-health, premature aging, heart disease, arthritis and stroke. These conditions tend to improve dramatically when the particular foci of infections are cleared with antimicrobials and anti-inflammatory agents. So that taking periodic doses of certain broad-spectrum antibiotics (tetracycline/sulfa drugs) help to prolong life by removing occult, focal infections in the body. According to E.M. Molnar M.D. "There have been several experiments which have shown that sulfa drugs, predecessors of antibiotics, can extend the life of laboratory animals, when given every day in small doses". A course of tetracycline or septrin plus flagyl every few months in the presence of focal disease will ensure good health and prolong life. Preferably, the administration of antibiotics should be preceded by culture and sensitivity testing. There is evidence that metronidazole (2g nightly for 3 consecutive nights every 3 months) dramatically improves symptoms of rheumatoid arthritis. Further, corroborative evidence comes from the jungles of South America where some primitive tribes who periodically consume a herb rich in tetracyclines live very long. From personal observation, I have discovered in my home town that lepers who took dapsone and other antimicrobials regularly for their affliction survived in good health longer than their non-leprous peers who did not take antimicrobials on a regular basis. Still on personal experience, I have discovered that following a course of co-trinoxazole or ofloxacin, I often feel a definite, unusual, physical upliftment and total rejuvenation. Readers, I exhort you to keep an open mind and try out the concept to see for yourself.

In a similar vein, the Russian pathologist Iliya Metchnikov (d. 1916), put forward the idea that man does not die or age naturally, but in fact poisons himself. Ill-health and senility are caused by auto-intoxication resulting from continuous putrefaction in the large intestine. This process is said to be arrested by the lactic-acid bacillus in sour milk or yoghurt. The proverbial longevity of Bulgarians is attributed to regular consumption of probiotics in yoghurt. Similarly, the regular consumption of probiotics and prebiotics protect against putrefaction in the large intestine to boost immunity and longevity. However, for fear of introducing antibiotic resistance, it may be more expedient to use herbal antimicrobial supplements such as garlic, onions, sweddish bitters, apple cider vinegar and dates to clean occult, foci infections to make for excellent health and longevity.

Smoking

Tobacco and snuff are definite anti-aphrodisiacs that destroy sexual potency. Indeed, it has been shown that there is a latent antagonism in the male body between tobacco and women, such that the taste for one diminishes the taste and capacity for the other. For this reason most people who want to retain their sexual potency into ripe old age should eschew smoking and chewing of tobacco. A famous physician once said, "Any man who smokes cigars and drinks soda water can sleep with my wife". So sure was he that such a man would be impotent.

REGULAR MEAL TIMES

One of the most important habits necessary for life-long vitality and eventual longevity is the habit of eating food at regular specified times of the day. This works out so well because the human body is itself a well-programmed machine that functions best in a highly organized fashion. This is especially true of the human digestive tract.

The indiscriminate shoveling of food down the digestive tract does not encourage optimal digestion and absorption. Instead, it encourages indigestion in the short term and more disabling diseases in the long term.

The result is often a miserable life that is punctuated by frequent ill-health which eventually culminates in premature aging and death.

Most people are used to eating three meals a day; in the morning, afternoon and evening. The trouble is that the intervals between meal times is often so staggered that one day, breakfast is at 7 am and the next day, it is taken at 10 am. Lunch for one day is at 12:30pm and the next day, it is taken at 4:30pm. Another person eats supper one evening at 6pm and the next day eats supper at 9:00pm. As far as these people are concerned, they have eaten 3 square meals in a day, regardless of what time the meals were shoveled down their stomachs. This is very unhealthy and nutritionally unwise.

The time variation for a particular meal must not exceed one hour. Breakfast time, for instance, should range from 7:30am to 8:30am; lunch time should fall between 1:30pm and 2:30pm; while supper should be between 6:30 and 7:30pm, daily. The variation of ½ - 1 hr is already quite liberal; the shorter the range the healthier. The ideal is to eat at the same time every day, by the hour and minute if possible. This ideal is of course impracticable for most people and hence the 1 hr variation.

There is a physiological reason why it is important to wait till the stomach is empty before shoveling in the next load of food. It is a known fact that as long as there is food in the stomach, movement along the entire length of the intestine is slowed down. But as soon as the stomach is empty, there is sudden upsurge in peristaltic activity in the small intestine. This squirts food from the small intestine through the ileocaecal valve into the large intestine. This arrangement is mediated through a reflex action called the "gastroileal" reflex. This affects the overall transit time of the intestinal tract. Indiscriminate feeding that does not give the stomach time to be completely empty tends to prolong the transit time leading to constipation and all its attendant sequelae, including cancer of the colon, appendicitis and so on.

The only certain way of telling that the stomach is empty and ready for the next load of food is through the "hunger pangs". It is very important to allow oneself to experience hunger-pangs before each meal. If you don't feel hungry, do not eat.

This is absolutely true for lunch and supper. Breakfast is of course necessary and routine and one does not need hunger pangs to dictate its timing.

For the average person, breakfast time should range from 7:30am to 8:30am. If, for instance, by 9:00am one has not eaten breakfast, it is best to forfeit it altogether and wait for lunch instead.

Lunch time should range from 1:30pm to 2:30pm, 5 hours after breakfast and this should be observed religiously for lifelong health and longevity. Within this range, one should observe the "hunger pangs" rule as strictly as possible. If by 1:30pm one is not feeling hungry, it is best to postpone lunch till 2:30pm when one feels really hungry enough to eat. And if by 2:30pm, you still do not feel like eating, it is far healthier to forego lunch altogether and wait for an earlier supper at about 6:30pm. This vital principle of healthful eating cannot be over-emphasized.

Supper for all people should fall between 6:30pm and 7:30pm, (i.e. 5 hours from lunch) and this should be observed religiously for total wellness. Here again it is wise to wait until one feels really hungry enough to eat. The lower limit of 7:30pm must however, be strictly observed for life-long health. No wise person would eat or drink anything after 7:30pm. Night-time is the resting period of the human digestive tract. Any violation spells ill-health the next day. This is so because the body systems are less efficient at night, there is a lot of production of waste matter which only goes to clog the system further to cause frequent irritating illnesses in the short-term and more serious diseases in the long term.

Meal-time rigidity may appear burdensome at first, but after a few days of drilling the stomach, the entire body systems easily adjust to the new and more natural schedule. The benefit is a life-time of vivacious living, full of zest and youthfulness into ripe old age.

One closing remark about supper is that it must be light always (brown rice and oatmeal). No place for heavy meals like pounded yam, amala, eba or tuwo. It is best to indulge in these heavy, high calorie meals at breakfast and lunch but never at supper. The only cereal meal allowed at supper is brown rice and oatmeal. The rice could be supplemented with fish pepper soup for palatability. The only other foods allowed as the permanent representative at every meal are fruits and vegetables. The reasons for eating only light meals at supper are two-fold: the first is that one is not likely to use up a lot of energy during sleep so that any excess will only go to form harmful fat; secondly, heavy meals just before bed time will interfere with sleep at night. The immediate result of eating heavy meals just before bed is that one wakes up next morning feeling drowsy, tired, irritable and unable to think or concentrate. Moreover, heavy meals at supper produce a lot of urine that forces a person to make frequent trips to the toilet. Heavy meals produce excess urine in two ways: first, following digestion and absorption, lots of waste products are produced which must be excreted at once through the urine. Secondly, eating a heavy meal usually goes along with drinking some liquid to help push it down. This liquid plus the natural water of the food all contribute to the formation of more urine at night leading to more frequent visit to the loo.

A light meal eaten early, not later than 7:30pm in the evening, however, needs little liquid to wash it down. Even when some liquid is taken early on in the evening, it is excreted before one finally retires, at about 9 - 10pm. This leaves one free to sleep peacefully through the night. Indeed, nature intends that no urine at all be voided throughout the night, so that any increased frequency of micturition more than once a night points to dietary indiscretion or more serious problems such as diseases of the kidneys, diabetes mellitus or prostatism.

DRY MEALS

It is a very wise counsel, indeed the old hygiene rule that says people should avoid drinking water or any other liquid during meals. There are several reasons for this, the most important being that excess liquid around meal times dilute the acid medium of the stomach thereby interfering with digestion. This often leads to indigestion, dyspepsia, and poor absorption of digested food.

CHAPTER 26
DIETOTHERAPY

The major import of a book like this is exposition of the preventive as well as curative properties of food for the benefit of mankind. Studies of different population groups across the world have provided information on the health benefits or otherwise of different diets or foods; and the compilation of those different experiences have formed the basis of the following dieto-therapy section. Even though the emphasis here is on prevention rather than cure, overwhelming evidence abound supporting the theory that a proper selection of food and drink can go a long way to prevent and control or revert most common ailments that trouble man. For those who already suffer from these diseases, a lot can be gained by way of amelioration or even complete cure through correct choice of food.

Some common conditions that are amenable to preventive and/or curative diets include the following: hypertension, coronary artery disease, chronic constipation, irritable bowel syndrome, common cold, some cancers of the gastrointestinal tract, inflammatory bowel disease, hyperlipidaemia, hemorrhoids, anal fissure, oesophageal reflux, appendicitis, gallbladder stones, skin disease, eye disease and obesity.

Hypertension

Hypertension or high blood pressure is a disease that afflicts about 10 – 15% of the general population. It is a major cause of disability and death, contributing a large percentage of all deaths attributed to natural causes in our society.

About 90 – 98% of all cases of hypertension do not have demonstrable organic cause. This type of hypertension is referred to as essential hypertension. It tends to run in families. That is to say, if one's father or mother dies of hypertension related causes, then the siblings have a high chance of becoming hypertensive.

In the last two decades or so, accumulated scientific evidence supports the theory that essential hypertension can be prevented through correct dieting and regular moderate exercise. For those who already suffer from the disease, it can be effectively controlled through correct eating and regular, moderate exercise. The best and healthiest exercise for the hypertensive is a brisk walk for 20 – 30 minutes every other day. It has relaxing effects on the whole body to lower blood pressure.

The main thrust of anti-hypertensive diet is the avoidance of salt and high-salt foods. This is based on the theory that high salt intake can worsen or predispose a person to getting hypertension. Another consideration is the need to avoid highly saturated fatty foods that may damage blood vessels and lead to hypertension. White sugar, and all sweetened foods can also predispose people to obesity which in turn can leads to hypertension.

For anyone who has high blood pressure or is predisposed to it, the following recommendations will go a long way to prevent and/or control the condition. The recommended diet is called a high fibre diet, where fruits and vegetables form the pillar of the diet with little protein and little or no added fat at all.

Dietary Approach to Stopping Hypertension (DASH)

1. Avoid white sugar and all sweetened foods.
2. Avoid all baked foods and manufactured foods such as cakes, biscuits, chocolates, sweets, ice-cream and beverages.
3. Avoid all soft drinks (drink plain water instead)
4. Cut down on all animal foods except fish, chicken, eggs, liver and bushmeat.
5. Avoid alcohol or drink only very little if at all.
6. Reduce milk and milk products (because of high content of salt and saturated fat)
7. Avoid all salted foods (bacon, salted margarine, and salted peanuts.)
8. Eat fish and fish oil at least 2 times a week.
9. Eat at least five vegetables daily.
10. Avoid powdered carbohydrate (semovita, white flour foods, alibo, eba, garri, amala)
11. Make beans the staple food of the family (cook correctly and eat at breakfast and lunch).
12. Eat liver once a week (at weekends only).
13. Eat at least one egg per day.
14. Take a brisk walk for 20 – 30 minutes every other day or every day of the week.
15. Take Brewer's yeast, wheat-germ, and vitamin C every day (the 3 musketeers of our supernutrition programme).
16. Take zinc supplements daily (15mg).
17. Take multivitamin and multi mineral tabs daily.
18. Eat small but frequently: every 2 hours by the clock by the odd number.

19.   Folic acid: daily dosing with folic acid prevents complication of hypertensions and prevents cancer of the cervix.

20.   Antioxidants: best consumed as part of fruits and vegetables daily (see TABS).

Research at St. Bartholomew's Hospital, London, estimated that avoiding salt intake could half the number of people needing drugs to reduce blood pressure and could reduce premature deaths by 40,000 people per year. Out of 100 Americans who took little or no salt in their daily diet, only one was found to have hypertension.

For good result, a hypertensive person or persons predisposed to it should adopt a diet of vegetable salad in the morning (TABS) and brown rice should be made the staple diet at lunch and dinner to the exclusion of most other carbohydrates, if possible.

A healthy eating pattern and lifestyle from the start are your best assurance for staying healthy and preventing diseases or at least slowing its course. The aim is to eat smartly to prevent and manage diseases throughout life. You eat to live and not live to eat.

The choices you make about food each day, along with physical activity, will affect your health and how you feel today, tomorrow and in the future.

Your life is filled with choices. Every day you make thousands of choices, many related to food. Some seem trivial; others are important; but as insignificant as it may appear, a single choice of food, if it's made over and over again over many days, months and years, can have a major or even catastrophic consequence for you and your family members in the long term.

The practical steps and flexible guidelines in this book will help you choose wisely the nutritious foods to match your own needs, preferences and lifestyle in order to change your life for the better. Eating for health is one of the wisest decisions you will ever make.

DIABETES MELLITUS

Diabetes mellitus, especially Type 2, like hypertension, tends to run in the family. Correct eating combined with regular moderate exercise can go a long way to prevent or control the condition. The dietary control of diabetes mellitus is especially relevant in Type 2 diabetes, those with glucose intolerance, prediabetes and metabolic syndrome.

1. Beans should be made the mainstay of the diet. This is because the fibre in beans has marked hypoglycemic and hypolipidaemic property.
2. Starchy carbohydrates: This includes yam, brown rice, acha, sweet potato, guineacorn, cocoyam and millet. Contrary to previous teaching, recent research has confirmed that far from being harmful, starchy carbohydrates are beneficial to diabetics because they release glucose slowly to the body thereby avoiding sudden increase in blood sugar that could lead to hyperinsulinaemia, weight gain and worsening of diabetes.
3. Avoid sweetened foods and white sugar as much as possible.
4. Avoid alcohol or take only little if at all.
5. Take vitamin C, wheat-germ, Brewer's yeast every day.
6. Take vitamin E (600 iu) to prevent diabetic complications such as eye disease.
7. Take appropriate supplements daily (cinnamon, turmeric, cordyceps, chitosan, alphabetic, wellwoman and wellman).

ARTHRITIS

Rheumatoid arthritis is an autoimmune disease. Regular consumption of fish and fish oil is said to be very helpful in reducing the incidence of acute attacks in rheumatoid arthritis. It works best when eaten with foods rich in vitamin C.

PEPTIC ULCER DISEASE.

For reasons not quite well understood, it has been found that regular consumption of fruits and vegetables help to control the symptoms of peptic dyspepsia. In fact, some people believe it can lead to eventual cure of peptic ulcer disease. I strongly support this view from personal experience. I was myself a victim of troublesome dyspepsia until I embarked on the life-long vitality diet thirty years ago. One week after starting on the diet, my dyspepsia disappeared and I have remained free of the symptoms ever since. The fruits and vegetables provide vitamin C that helps in ulcer healing. A scientific study has found that 42% of peptic ulcer victims are deficient in vitamin C.

For maximum benefit however, one should combine the life-long vitality diet with regular moderate exercise which tones up the gut wall and prevents recurrence of the ulcers. Alcohol intake must be reduced or best avoided altogether. White sugar, chocolate and all sweetened foods and junk foods must be avoided completely to ensure long-term remission. Specifically one should avoid cassava and cassava products like "gari" completely. As stated in an earlier chapter, a study in India has found that peptic ulcer disease is restricted to Southern states that subsist on cassava products as their staple food. Another study from Ibadan Nigeria has shown that cassava and cassava products together constitute singular most important cause of peptic ulcer exacerbation in our environment.

THE COMMON COLD OR CATARRH

The daily consumption of plenty of fruits and vegetables protects one from frequent attacks of catarrh. This is again corroborated by personal experience. I have been virtually free from attacks of catarrh for many years even when everybody else is down with the ailment, especially during the harmattan season. No matter the degree of coldness of the ambient temperature, I take my bath with cold water and remain catarrh free.

The protective effect of fruits and vegetables against catarrh is again attributed to their high vitamin C content. This is indeed another example of an apple a day keeping the doctor away.

One cannot conclude properly on this subject of vitamin C and the common cold without mentioning the name of the legend Professor Linus Pauling of California, USA, twice Nobel Laureate, who had devoted much of his research work to proving the protective effect of vitamin C against the common cold. Professor Linus Pauling recommends a minimum of 2000mg of the vitamin per day for prevention of the common cold. An even higher dose is said to be a panacea for several other diseases, though it is yet to become a general medical opinion.

IRRITABLE BOWEL SYNDROME (IBS)

This is a disease condition in which a person's bowels are hypersensitive and change frequently from extreme constipation, with bead-like dark stools, to recurrent watery diarrhea. The patient is usually pre-occupied with his or her bowel movements. There's almost always an underlying emotional problem such as anxiety or neurosis. Eating foods rich in fruits and vegetables usually control the problem within a few weeks. The effect is even more dramatic when the diet is combined with moderate exercise and early morning drinking of 1.5litres of plain water on waking (water therapy).

CANCER

Total dietary calorie restriction or specifically limiting high calorie carbohydrates in the diet by reducing or eliminating powdered root starch (e.g. Amala, garri, alibo, semovita), saturated fat and red meat has been shown to reduce the incidence of certain tumours in mice and rats. By contrast, limiting the protein content of the diet generally had very little effect on the overall incidence of these tumours.

Both the quantity and the quality of dietary fat can influence tumour incidence or cancer. For instance cancer of the colon has been linked to a diet that is high in saturated fat and low in fibre – the typical diet of Western industrialized countries. Eating foods that are rich in fibre such as beans, fruits, vegetables and cereals has been linked to low incidence of cancers of the colon and rectum. This is based largely on comparative studies of the incidence of the disease in populations that eat unprocessed foods in rural African societies and those that eat highly processed low-fibre foods in developed societies like America and Britain. Unprocessed foods shorten intestinal transit time and prevent long stasis of faeces in the colon and rectum thereby discouraging the formation of toxic substances that cause cancer.

STEPS TO AVOIDING CANCER

1.	Avoid fried and smoked foods (including suya and fried chicken)
2.	Avoid smoking
3.	Boost the body's antioxidant and immune system
➢	Eat fruits and vegetables (5 – 8 servings per day)
➢	Eat high fibre, low– fat, and low protein diet
➢	Take nutritional supplements and antioxidants (they prevent cancer and often reverse pre-cancerous conditions)
➢	Take vitamin C daily
➢	Take vitamin A regularly.
➢	Take vitamin E
➢	Take multimineral and multivitamin supplement.
4.	Eat natural fats (including natural butter sparingly) in order to absorb vitamins A, D and E that are responsible for cancer prevention, healthy eyesight, bone strength, mental health and cardiovascular health.

HAEMORRHOIDS OR PILES

The consumption of refined and processed foods causes constipation. Constipation causes hard stools that are usually evacuated with straining defection. Such frequent straining encourages the formation of haemorrhoids or piles, especially, in sedentary office-workers. A change of diet to one that includes plenty of fruits and vegetables will prevent or dramatically control the problem of piles and other anorectal diseases. The effects are even more dramatic when the diet is combined with moderate exercise.

VARICOSE VEINS

Varicose veins are etiologically related to haermorrhoids or piles. They are common in persons who eat lots of sweet and/or refined foods like white flour, biscuits, chocolates and so on. A change of diet to fruits and vegetables combined with regular moderate regular exercise will go a long way to mitigate or even cure the condition altogether.

INFLAMMATORY BOWEL DISEASE

The incidence of chronic bowel disease and ulcerative colitis remain very low in most rural African populations because of the high fibre content of their diet. Unless the younger African generations stick to eating fresh, unprocessed cereals and vegetable diets like their ancestors, they will soon become victims of inflammatory bowel disease like people of the west who eat highly refined foods routinely.

CORONARY ARTERY DISEASE

Coronary artery disease, or CAD for short, is the greatest killer disease in western societies. It usually manifests most dramatically as heart attack and sudden death. The disease is beginning to rear its ugly head in developing countries like Nigeria, especially among our more affluent compatriots who ignorantly adopt western diet in the name of sophistication.

In order to forestall and reverse this ugly trend, our young ones must be tutored on the crucial need to avoid refined and processed foods including white sugar, amala, alibo, garri and all flour. They should instead be encouraged to stick to fresh, natural "straight-from-the-farm" foods. They should at the same time eat very little palm oil, no palm kernel oil and eat little coconut oil. They must also be told to avoid saturated fatty foods such as pork, liver, milk, milk products and red meat. Last but not the least important, they should be encouraged to eat fish regularly as this lowers the level of harmful cholesterol in the blood. This leaves the heart and blood vessels free of harmful atheromatous substances that usually cause premature ageing, heart attacks, sudden deaths or strokes.

For all-round protection and life-long vitality, the diet should be combined with regular moderate exercise.

HYPERLIPIDAEMIA

This is a group of diseases caused by an individual's inherent inability to handle lipid or fat metabolism. The result is an unhealthy accumulation of certain products of lipids in the blood. This can lead to premature aging of the blood vessels which in turn result in diseases like hypertension, heart attacks, and strokes.

A high fibre diet (such as TABS and TAMS) has the capability of lowering the raised level of harmful lipid metabolites in blood through a mechanism that is not yet fully understood. The foods capable of lowering blood lipid include fruits, vegetables, oatmeal, brown rice, guineacorn, millet and legumes, especially beans. You will notice that all these foods are conspicuously represented in the super nutrition diet recommended in this book.

ANAL FISSURE

Anal fissure are cracks in the lining of the anus which give rise to excruciating pain during defecation. The condition is most commonly found in people who pass stool frequently and those whose stools are usually hard (constipated). A change in diet to high fibre foods, rich in vegetables, fruits, oatmeal, brown rice, guineacorn, millet and beans usually promptly reverses the situation.

OESOPHAGEAL REFLUX (GERD)

For reasons not quite well understood, symptoms of oesophageal reflux or hiatus hernia are usually relieved by high fibre foods. Symptoms include heartburn and chest pain that worsen on stooping or lying flat and improve on sitting up in bed.

The reason may have to do with the fact that high fibre foods help to tone up the muscles of the gut wall which in turn improves the sphincteric function of the cardio-oesophageal junction. The improvement of symptoms is most impressive when the high fibre foods are combined with regular moderate exercise. The simple addition of fibre supplements (psyllium) to your meals is very important and may actually cure the condition. Taking plenty of water 30 minutes before meals is also very important.

APPENDICITIS

Appendicitis is more common in people who eat refined western type of diet, especially bread, biscuits, chocolates and similar junk foods. Conversely, appendicitis is rare in people who eat mainly traditional African diets which include unprocessed cereals, fruits and vegetables.

As an insurance against appendicitis, therefore, people should avoid refined foods such as sugar, bread, flour, biscuits, sweets and chocolates. They should, instead, eat fresh, wholesome, unprocessed, "straight-from-the-farm" foods always.

GALLBLADDER STONES

This is another disease that is common in western countries but is rare in rural African societies. The epidemiological difference is once again ascribed to the high fibre diet of the rural African which tends to protect against gallbladder stones through a mechanism that is not yet well understood.

SKIN DISEASES

Regular consumption of fruits and vegetables leads to a healthy skin due to the high level of vitamin A and C in these foods. If you add healthy oils like olive oil to fruits and vegetables as in TAMS and TABS, your skin will be so clear and healthy that you will not have to spend money on skin moisturizer and similar cosmetics for the rest of your life.

EYE DISEASES

The diet advocated in this book has a very high level of vitamin A and riboflavin which helps to keep the eyes clear and disease resistant. This is further improved by regular consumption of Brewer's yeast which contains about 16 minerals and vitamins.

OBESITY AND WEIGHT REDUCTION

For reasons not yet understood, high dietary fibre tends to promote weight loss in people who are overweight. The reason for the weight reducing property of fibre include the low-calorie content of fibre foods and the feelings of satiety that prevents from indulging high calorie foods.

For rapid weight reduction, the high fibre diet must be combined with regular exercise in the form of "brisk walk" for 45 minutes a day from 6:00am to 6:45am before breakfast daily for at least 5 days a week. For an even more rapid weight reduction, eat according to your blood group as advocated elsewhere in this book.

According to Dr. Newburg of Michigan University in the USA, even the extremely fat person can reduce to normal weight and glandular functions returned to normal simply through a carefully selected diet without glandular or hormonal therapy. For permanent weight loss, eating plenty of protein foods (beans, bambara nuts, lima beans, soya beans) at breakfast is the best slendering food because of their high specific dynamic action. For gradual, sustained, weight loss one should take at least one pint of fat-free yoghurt daily as this staves off hunger pangs for long periods in addition to providing high quality nutrients.

Obesity is defined as a BMI greater than 30. Central obesity is even more dangerous than generalized obesity. Central obesity or "pot-belly" is measured by taking waist-hip ratio.

In the clinic setting, the most practical means of assessing obesity is by the use of Skinfold Calipers over the triceps muscle. The measurement should be done equidistant from the tip of the acromion and the olecranon process.

COMPLICATIONS OF OBESITY:

1. Psychological: Obesity creates emotional problems such as neurosis and disturbance about body image, especially in those whose obesity started in early adolescence.

2. Mechanical disability: Apart from aesthetic considerations, obesity leads to mechanical disabilities, predisposing to metabolic and cardiovascular disorders and so reduces life expectancy drastically. Excess weight leads to flat feet and osteoarthritis of the knees, hips and lumbar spine. Excess weight in the abdomen leads to abdominal hernias and varicose veins. Adipose tissue around the chest and under the diaphragm interferes with respiration and predisposes to bronchitis and non-cardiac dyspnoea on exertion.

3. Diabetes Mellitus: Adult onset diabetes mellitus is more common in obese persons.

4. Hypercholesterolaemia and gallbladder stones are more common in obese persons.

5. Hypertension is more in obese persons and when they lose weight their blood pressure falls.

6. Hypercholesterolaemia coupled with hypertension makes coronary heart disease very common in obese persons.

7. Respiratory complications: Difficulty with breathing along with somnolence, the so-called; "Pickwickian syndrome".

8. Skin: Skin infections are more common in obese people.

9. Life Expectancy: it has been shown that a 45year old man whose body weight is 12kg above the standard weight for his age reduces his life expectancy by 25%. In other words, if the contemporaries of the person in question who are of normal weight are to live for 100 years, the over-weight

person would not exceed 75 years. The risks of obesity in women are less than in men. A regular practice of weighing patients and examining them for evidence of excessive fat would prevent overlooking obesity as a cause of so many disease conditions. This is a wake-up call for all doctors and health workers who examine and diagnose diseases in patients.

TREATMENT OF OBESITY

The essence of treatment is to reduce the energy content of the person's diet. Based on food composition tables, 100g of cereals supplies 1.5MJ of energy whereas starch carbohydrates like yam, sweet potatoes and cocoyam only provide 0.5MJ per 100g. This is the food for slimmers and those who want to maintain their body weight. They should avoid high energy foods like amala, garri, alibo, tuwo, fufu and semovita.

Another dietetic principle for rapid weight loss is the concept of eating according to blood groups. This enables clients lose weight rapidily over a few months.

Weight loss can also be facilitated by consuming calcium-rich foods like locust beans and baobab leaves. To further accelerate the rate of weight loss, the client should avoid junk foods, deep-fried foods, soft drinks, red meat and oestrogenic foods.

When obese persons adopt the above strategies and add to it fasting for the first 3-days of every month, the weight loss becomes rapid and permanent.

POT BELLY EPIDEMIC

As a consequence of the increasing obesity in the world including developing countries like Nigeria, we are seeing a lot of potbellied men across the nation – the so-called "pregnant men". The problem is appropriately a manifestation of middle-life obesity, the type of obesity associated with the worst health outcome.

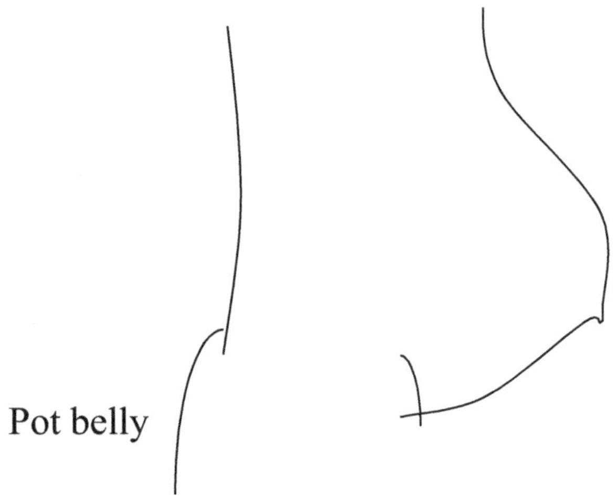

Pot belly

The commonest underlying metabolic disorder associated with this type of obesity is low -free testosteronein the body. The features of which include:

a.   Decreased libido
b.   Brain fag
c.   Fewer erections on waking.
d.   Erectile dysfunction.
e.   Impotence
f.   Persistent fatigue
g.   Decreased sense of well being
h.   Insomnia.

Even though pot-belly is associated with middle-age (the so-called andropause), the above signs of low free testosterone are being seen with high frequency in men as young as 30 years due to the high rate of pollutants present in foodstuffs, air and drugs. This has led to an unexpected high incidence of erectile dysfunctions in these young people manifestating in early divorce in our society.

Management of Pot-Belly: This is similar to the management of generalized obesity with the following particulars:

1.   Exercise – increase physical exercise to 2hours per week
2.   Fasting – water fasting for the first 3 days of every calendar month detoxifies the body as well as decreases the level of hyper insulinaemia that encourages weight gain in middle-age.
3.   Avoid fried, junk and fast foods
4.   Avoid alcohol
5.   Eat according to blood group
6.   Avoid estrogenic foods (soya beans, products, cabbage, millet, trans-fats, small leaved spinach).
7.   Eat only anti-estrogenic foods. Examples of anti-estrogenic (belly-bursting) foods include:
(a)   Apples (eat peeled at bed time)
(b)   Green beans (eat with rice at lunch or dinner)
(c)   Beetroot and beetroot leaves
(d)   Carrots (Miracle juice)
(e)   Grapefruit (drink as part of the 3-day monthly fruit-fasts or as Sabbath fast)

(f)   Lemon juice drink in water (30minutes before and 30 minutes after meals daily to alkalinize the whole body to facilitate weight loss)

(g)   Onion - eat one whole medium onion daily

(h)   Radish – eat with lunch or dinner

(i)   Spinach

(j)   Tomatoes

(k)   Watermelon and watermelon seeds

INSOMNIA

According to Williams Shakespare, "Depression is that which taketh away thy stomach, thy pleasure and thy golden sleep".

Insomnia refers to the inability of a person to fall asleep or sleep through the night in the absence of an identifiable cause.

Sleep is the providential prescription for a tired body. After a hard day's job, it is very important that one gets a good restful sleep at night. The remedy for tired limbs and eyes is not another cup of tea or coffee; neither is the problem solved by swallowing two tablets of "panadol" or "aspirin"; the cure is simply a "good sleep" that leaves one feeling refreshed and rejuvenated the next morning.

Tiredness is brought on by the accumulation of certain products of metabolism such as lactic acid, in the body. When one sleeps, these products are slowly "burnt up" by aerobic respiration to form water and carbon dioxide, which are then promptly excreted. No drug can take the place of a golden sleep in the relief of tiredness. If one wakes up still feeling tired and unrefreshed after an apparently adequate time in bed, then it is a sign of poor sleep. The reason may range from simple causes like a heavy meal just before bed or going to bed either too early or too late. Other less common but more serious causes of poor sleep include organic or psychiatric disorders.

On how much sleep is adequate for any individual person, the old teaching used to be   that it varies from person to person. That some people need fewer hours of sleep to get refreshed, while others require more hours of sleep in order to feel refreshed in the morning. That as long as one wakes up feeling alert and rejuvenated the next morning, one can assume he or she has had good sleep at night. But more recent scientific research has discovered that people on average require about 7 to 8 hours of sleep at night for optimum health. Those who slept for less than 7 hours at night tended to have higher blood pressures than those who slept for 7 to 8 hours. And those who slept for longer than 8 hours also had higher blood pressures than those who slept 7 – 8 hours per night. I personally documented this in a survey I carried out in a sample population of otherwise healthy people living in a ward in Kaduna metropolis. This formed part of my dissertation for the MBBS degree at the Ahmadu Bello University Medical School, Zaria, in June 1981. I was very pleased to read in a foreign medical journal a few years later that similar findings were independently documented somewhere in California, in the USA.

To sleep for 7 to 8hours at night, it is crucial for one to go to bed at regular times (9:00 to 10:00pm) in the evenings and to observe this strictly every night. This will enable one's body to adjust and anticipate sleep. I personally discovered that for a good night's sleep, I need to be in bed around 10:00pm; I usually then wake up around 5:30am feeling refreshed and alert after 7 ½ hours' sleep every night. If I go to bed later than 11pm, I usually wake up feeling unrefreshed and this usually spoils my whole day. If on the other hand I retire earlier, say by 8.00pm, I invariably have to wake around 12.00midnight – 2am, then sleep again from 3.00-5.30 am

The following tips will help improve sleep in people with non-organic sleep disorders:

➢ Regularization of bed time
➢ The use of bedroom strictly for sleep and sexual activities
➢ Regular moderate exercise, at least 3-4 times a week, interspersed with weight training and weight lifting two times a week is almost magical.
➢ Avoidance of alcohol and caffeine
➢ Reduction of fluid intake after 7:30pm
➢ Avoidance of meals after 7:30pm

I have personally discovered that a brisk 10 minutes' walk in fresh air a few minutes before bed or 50 press-ups 2 hours before bedtime at 8:00pm is about the best hypnotic for those with persistent sleep disorders. If for any reason one cannot sleep throughout the night, it is alright to break sleep into phases like say from 7:30 pm to 9:30 pm then meet with family or friends to discuss and share pleasantries till 12:00 midnight then resume sleep till 5:30 am. This brings the total numbers of hours of sleep to 7 ½ hrs which is quite okay. Finally, if sleep refuses to come, do not sit up and do not leave your bed and walk around the house but simply remain horizontal in bed and pick a book and read while lying flat in bed. The body will count it as part of your rest period.

HAPPY FOODS AND SAD FOODS

Happy Foods

Foods which contain the amino acid tryptophan, tyrosine and the B complex vitamins are said to be "happy foods" because they elevate mood when taken along with carbohydrate. When you add folic acid (1 daily) and vitamin C (500mg twice daily) to these happy foods, dopamine is produced which elevates mood. These happy foods are already integral and bonafide members of TABS and TAMS. These foods include:

1.   Chicken chest, Turkey, Cottage cheese (for tryptophan)
2.   Fresh meat, yoghurt, milk (for tyrosine)
3.   Liver, kidney, heart, Brewer's yeast, green leaves, fish, brown rice and
4.   wheat germ (for vitamin B complex)
5.   Vitamin F: is a collection of unsaturated fatty acids, linolenic, linoleic and arachidonic acid. They are also called "essential fatty acids" (EFA). Vitamin F improves mood through its activities on the central nervous system and the endocrine glands. Foods rich in vitamin F include wheat-germ, corn or maize oil and tree nuts (such as almonds, walnuts and cashew nuts).
6.   Vitamin D: in addition to the regulation of absorption of calcium and phosphorous, vitamin D, also strengthens and stabilizes the central nervous system and positively affects the activity of the thyroid gland. Weekly cod liver oil supplementation may be all that is needed to replenish the stores of this vitamin, especially in office workers who are always well-wrapped up and remain shaded from sun light throughout the period they are in their offices or airconditioned cars. Regular bathing with soaps also interferes with the ability of the skin to form vitamin D from sunshine. This is another reason why vitamin D deficiency may be very common in sophisticated towns where we have people who rarely get exposed to sunshine and at the same time use lots of soap frequently, morning and evening daily.

Happy foods are best eaten in the mornings to help brightens one's day. TABS with its dressing and high quality protein are a happy meal par excellence for daily consumption.

Sad Foods

Sad foods depress the mood because of their physiological properties. These foods include sugar, chocolate, high fat foods like mayonnaise and marbled meat. Other sad foods include lentils, cabbage, soyamilk, and other soya products and chickpeas (hummus). They are sad foods because they inhibit the thyroid gland. Another food item that is a very "sad food" is the seasoning agent monosodium glutamate (MSG). It causes headaches, dizziness and other unpleasant feelings and has been associated with depression. Glutamate in MSG releases sugar from the liver and makes it unavailable when needed for active work, thereby causing fatigue and general body weakness.

Alcohol is also a very sad food because it depresses the central nervous system. The practice of washing down lunch with beer or other alcoholic beverages is most unhealthy and only helps to spoil the rest of one's day.

CHAPTER 27
PREGNANCY AND NUTRITION

ANTENATAL NUTRITION

The development of any country depends on its people and the quality of the people in turn depends on the I.Q. of the individuals in the population. If Nigeria is to progress developmentally to compete in the global arena, we must work hard to produce high quality citizens with high average I.Q. to rebrand this country and to take it to the level of an industrialized nation. Women of child bearing age and pregnant women must be fed well and correctly to ensure that the brains of future generations of Nigerians are well-developed.

The quantity and quality of food a woman eats during pregnancy can affect the outcome of her pregnancy in several ways. For instance, lack of certain vitamins can cause deficiency diseases in the infant while too much of some nutrients can affect the newborn child adversely. It is therefore vital for pregnant mothers to eat sensibly in order to have healthy mother and child at confinement. Furthermore, recent research findings suggest that the life expectancy of a newborn infant at birth is pre-determined by the mother's diet while she was pregnant with the child. It has been proven that the seed of diseases such as high blood pressure and diabetes mellitus are sown in the womb, even though these diseases do not manifest until early or late adulthood.

For a clear understanding of this most important topic of antenatal nutrition therefore, I wish to discuss it in relation to the various classes of food mentioned earlier in the book.

There are no "special diets" for pregnancy, nor are there any particular foods that must be taken. This is because a lot of adaptive changes take place in the pregnant woman to minimize the requirements for protein, iron and calcium. Nevertheless, there are certain general advices and recommendations that will help improve the overall health of both mother and baby.

CARBOHYDRATES AND PREGNANCY

The quantity of carbohydrate allowed a pregnant woman is predicated on her pre-pregnancy body weight. If she is generally an obese woman before pregnancy, it is advised that she continues to eat normally throughout pregnancy and confinement. This is because calorie restriction in an obese pregnant woman (BMI >30) is detrimental to the growing fetus in her body. But if she eats normally, even if she gains more weight during the pregnancy, her fetus is protected and will grow normally to a healthy infant at birth.

For a woman with average body weight before pregnancy (BMI<29), the amount of food (refined/processed carbohydrate and fat) should be restricted to prevent large baby syndrome.

For underweight pregnant women, there is a need to increase food intake during pregnancyin order to reduce the incidence of low-birth weight babies at delivery.

In order to determine the weight status of a woman, one should calculate the body mass index (BMI) of the woman using her pre-pregnancy body weight. This is done by dividing the pre-pregnancy weight of the woman (kg) by the square of her height (in metres). If the BMI of the woman is less than 18.5, then she is underweight and must be encouraged to eat a lot more especially protein to improve the outcome of her pregnancy. If the BMI falls within 18.5-24.9, then the woman is of average body build and she should be told to restrict eating refined carbohydrate and saturated fats to prevent large baby syndrome. For overweight and obese women with BMI greater than 25, they should eat normally because even if they gain more weight, it will not affect their unborn baby.

Weight gain during pregnancy is a very sensitive index of the general well-being of a pregnant woman. The average weight gained is around 3.5kg by the 20th week of gestation and 0.5kg per week for rest of the pregnancy. Any significant deviation from this average requires thorough investigation. Excessive weight gain is worse than poor or no weight gain. Considering the serious medical implications that excessive weight gain portends, such weight-gain may not be lost completely after delivery and with successive pregnancies, frank obesity may develop with its harmful effects. It is therefore very important for women to try and lose all excess weight gained with each pregnancy before the next pregnancy in order to prevent future obesity and its sequelae.

PROTEIN AND PREGNANCY

As mentioned earlier, protein is the building block of the human body. This means that a pregnant woman carrying a growing child requires adequate protein intake to ensure a favourable pregnancy outcome, no matter her pre-pregnancy status. A pregnant woman requires at least 0.9g/kg body weight of protein, per day for the fetus to grow well, compared with 0.5g/kg body weight for non-pregnant women.

Moreover, recent research has shown that adequate protein intake in early pregnancy reduces the incidence of the dreaded disease called "toxaemia of pregnancy", which is one of the major causes of maternal morbidity and mortality all over the world. A high protein diet is highly recommended for women predisposed to getting toxaemia of pregnancy especially for primiparous women, women with history of toxaemia of pregnancy and the hypertensive pregnant woman. These should include at least two eggs per day, some lean meat daily, beans, soya milk, or soya products, milk, cheese, yoghurt, nuts, Brewer's yeast and fish. For those who can afford it, the best means of meeting protein needs in pregnancy is to take at least ½ cup of powdered skimmed milk unless precluded by blood group incompatibility.

The beneficial effect of a high protein diet has been attributed to the high content of zinc in these foods. Research has also shown that zinc deficiency causes pregnancy complications such as fetal growth retardation and pre-eclamptic toxaemia of pregnancy.

FATS AND OILS IN PREGNANCY

For best pregnancy outcomes, both for mother and child, the pregnant woman is encouraged to eat little oily fish (sardine, mackerel and herring) 2 to 3 times a week. If fish is difficult to come by, the pregnant mother may take cod liver oil (mercury-free) from "SEVEN SEAS" two (2) times a week. These oils are particularly good for brain development of the foetus. Other sources of healthy fats in pregnancy include: tree nuts such as walnuts, almond and cashew nuts as well as seed oils like sesame, sunflower and flaxseed oils.

For the sake of emphasis, pregnant women should avoid fried foods and particularly processed fast-foods that are loaded with saturated oils and trans-fats as these may likely sow the seeds of chronic diseases like hypertension, diabetes and cancer in the child. They should therefore, avoid all manufactured or factory processed foods and instead go for fresh unprocessed straight-from-the-farm starch and grain foods that are boiled not fried.

MINERALS AND PREGNANCY

(a)   **Iron**:   Iron is the major element required for blood formation. The requirement for iron increases during pregnancy, and especially during the second half of gestation. It was therefore conventional to give oral iron supplementation routinely throughout pregnancy.

But more recent research has demonstrated that orally administered iron impairs the absorption of other vital elements needed by the fetus, especially vitamin F and the mineral zinc. It is therefore currently advised that unless a woman is proven to be iron deficient, supported by laboratory test, iron supplementation should be withheld until the second half of the pregnancy and even then only a small prophylactic dose should be given and not treatment doses.

Iron deficiency anaemia is common in pregnancy because of increased demand for iron by the growing fetus. Iron rich foods should be taken regularly during pregnancy. These foods include beans, eggs, liver, red meat, bushmeat, fruits and vegetables. Routine 'blood' examination to check for the level of haemoglobin in all pregnant women is vital. For women whose haemoglobin is less than 12g/dl, iron supplementation should be given from the beginning of antenatal care. For those above 12g/dl, one can afford to wait till the second trimester to begin iron supplementation.

(b)   **Calcium:** In view of the abundant sunshine in the tropics, calcium deficiency is not common and therefore routine calcium supplementation is not generally advised. The exceptions are women who are always in-doors and who even when they are outdoors, remain fully clad, thereby preventing sunshine from reaching their skins. These women will benefit from vitamin D (100 iu/day) and calcium supplementation during pregnancy. Another important group of women that require calcium supplementation are those who are predisposed to toxaemia of pregnancy. Calcium carbonate, given 2g per day, is said to prevent toxaemia of pregnancy.

The best way to meet the extra calcium needs in pregnancy is to increase powdered milk intake to about ½ a litre per day at least. In an environment where milk is beyond the affordability of most families, the most convenient sources of calcium are green leafy vegetables, fish bones, mazarkwaila, chicken bones, egusi and beans. Locust beans (dadawa), baobab leaves (miyan kuka) and beniseed are excellent sources of calcium in our environment. Adding apple cider vinegar to Dr. Affi's Breakfast Salad boosts calcium absorption.

(c)   **Zinc:**   Animal studies have shown that zinc deficiency may cause pregnancy complications such as pre-eclampsia and fetal growth retardation. Unfortunately, zinc supplementation does not appear to help the situation. The answer may lie in withholding oral iron supplementation during the first half of pregnancy, unless specifically indicated. Another approach is to encourage high protein diet that supplies adequate absorbable zinc throughout pregnancy (eggs, milk, fish, lean meat, milk, yoghurt, bambara nuts, beans, cheese).

(d) **Iodine:** Where endemic goiter is common, injecting pregnant women intramuscularly with iodized oil once every three years reduces the risk of cretinous children. In addition, iodized salt should be used for cooking always but only in populations with demonstrable iodine deficiency. Sea salt (Brittany Brand) is highly recommended.

VITAMINS AND PREGNANCY

Unless a deficiency in a particular vitamin is clearly demonstrated, unsupervised taking of multi-vitamins during pregnancy is not recommended. This is because some vitamins are potentially teratogenic, meaning they can cause congenital abnormalities in the infant. For instance, excessive consumption of vitamin A during the second month of pregnancy causes congenital malformation, including absent ears, cleft palate, cortical blindness, congenital heart disease and abnormalities of the central nervous system.

The only vitamin that has been shown to be consistently low in malnourished pregnant women is folic acid. It is therefore the only vitamin that may be prescribed routinely to all pregnant women. Folic acid deficiency has been linked with pregnancy complications such as pre-eclampsia and abruptio placentae; although this has not been unequivocally proved. There is also a strong argument supporting the theory that the deficiency of folic acid causes malformation of the central nervous system including spina bifida.

The recommended routine prophylactic dose of folic acid throughout pregnancy is 200-400mcg per day. However, if there is established nutritional anaemia, the dose should be increased to a minimum of 1000mcg/day (i.e. 400mcg taken three times a day).

In pregnancy, if a good mixed diet is eaten there is no need to prescribe any vitamin supplements. If there is any doubt about the quality of the diet, as is the case in most families in the country today, however, it is most desirable for all pregnant women to be placed on vitamins B complex, vitamin D and folic acid supplementation. Supplementation should be routine prior to and during all pregnancies. Folic acid and vitamin B complex before pregnancy helps prevent certain complications in pregnancy such as spina bifida, recurrent abortions, premature labour and still-births.

Taking into consideration the poor nutritional status of our people, some pharmaceutical companies have produced proprietary multivitamins and multimineral supplements which have proved useful for the average pregnant woman in our society. In our practice, PREGNACARE has proved useful in the Nigerian environment.

In conclusion, some women develop bizarre appetites such as pica during pregnancy. Such bizarre appetites are not unusual in pregnancy so that simple explanations often effectively control such abnormal behavior.

For good health, a mother who is breastfeeding her baby must eat an adequate diet. This is highly desirable to meet the need for extra calories for the baby. A diet of brown rice and beans with fish or eggs is adequate. With slight modification to suit the pregnancy state and lactation, the TABS and TAMS are applicable to these women.

CHAPTER 28
INFANT AND CHILD NUTRITION

"Degeneration and other senile diseases begin in early life, resulting from over-nourishment in infancy through childhood, adolescence and adulthood."

(Hywel Davies)

INFANT NUTRITION

Nutrition in infancy and childhood is very critical in the sense that any significant aberration can leave permanent irrepairable damage right into adulthood. According to Marilyn and Sarah, "Junk foods make junk children". Lactation is not fully established for the first 2 or 3 days of the birth of a baby, and during this short period of partial starvation, an infant derives much of his energy from a large store of glycogen in the liver. The glycogen content of the liver in a full term infant at birth is about 100g/kg. It falls to the normal adult level of about 20 g/kg by the end of the first week.

For the new born infant, the best food is the mother's breast milk. This alone is sufficient to sustain the child up to the age of 6 months. For the first 6 months of life, there is no need for any extra feeds, not even water. Even in the hottest part of the world, research has shown that the new born infant up to the age of 6 months does not need extra plain water. The water in breast milk is adequate for normal growth and health. During these first 6 months of life, the child does not require any proprietary glucose or multivitamins. Breast milk supplies all the necessary nutrients for optimal growth during these early months of life. However, for the breast feeding to be satisfactory`, it must be frequent and on demand. Premature infants and those with low birth weight, however, do require earlier food supplementation at 2-3 months. For instance, they require early iron supplementation in view of their low iron stores which soon gets exhausted by the end of the second month of life. This earlier supplementation should be around the end of the second month postnatal.

For normal term infants, it is recommended that solid food supplementation should start at the beginning of the 6th month of life and should be completed by the end of the sixth month postnatal. In order words, by the end of the 6th month of age, the child should be on soft family diet. Solid foods are necessary to supply the much needed iron for growth and good mental performance in school later in life. Timely and correct food supplementation at this stage is very crucial because if not properly done, a child can easily be tipped into anaemia as iron stores acquired from the mother during pregnancy gets exhausted by the 3rd to 4th month of life. Furthermore, for most babies, if not properly supplemented at this stage, the anaemia so precipitated tends to persist throughout childhood. This persistent anaemia of childhood has been shown to adversely affect a child's performance in school. The anaemia so acquired is usually perpetuated or worsened by worm infestations acquired at 7-10 months when a child crawls around eating pica and similar dirt. This can be helped by regular de-worming with anti-helmintics from age of 7months. Regular de-worming using any of the common anti-helmintics at 4 monthly intervals is adequate, but I have personally found Zentel to be particularly useful.

To further improve the iron stores of a child, food supplementation during weaning should be with iron–rich pap using red guinea corn and millet rather than maize pap because guinea corn is richer in iron than maize. The pap should be made very thick with added mazankwaila, olive oil, egg, avocado, dessicated liver and Brewer's yeast to improve the nutritional value of the supplement. All these items can be added while the pap is on fire.

From the foregoing discussion on infant and child nutrition, you would have noticed that I have not mentioned anything about infant formula.

Infant formulas must never be used to feed children unless the mother cannot breastfeed for a definite reason such as maternal death or infection (eg.HIV positivity or tuberculosis). Infant formulas are first and foremost, too expensive for most mothers. Moreover, cow's milk predisposes some children to diseases such as eczema, asthma, vitamin C deficiency and some yet unveiled conditions, both physical and psychological.

Breast milk, on the other hand, protects children against several important childhood diseases like diarrhea, chest infection and skin diseases. In God's providential plan for the human child, there is no place for the use of cow's milk to feed the human child. No amount of high technology or civilization can change that. Even after the child has been weaned on to the family diet, breastfeeding should continue for about a year or two. This is healthy for both mother and child, physically and psychologically for balanced emotional development of the child.

As mentioned above, human breastmilk is the best feed for the human infant. The advantages of breastfeeding over bottle feeding with cow's milk are as follows:

a. Human milk contains several host resistance factors such as anti staphylococcal factor, secretory IgA and other immunoglobulins, and lysozymes.

b. Breast milk is hygienic and always ready.

c. Breast feeding encourage's mother-child psychological bonding.

d. Human milk contains lactogerm which inhibits disease-causing intestinal microorganism.

e. Breast fed babies are at a reduced risk of neonatal tetany, hypertonic dehydration, infant obesity, allergy to cow's milk and certain other hazards yet unknown.

f. Artificially fed babies are often bigger than breast fed babies and this is thought to be linked to shorter life expectancy in formula-fed children. The extra-weight is adaptation to the artificial food in the first months of life which may very well sow the seed of certain disorders of later life including hypertension and allergies.

In view of the above litany of problems, bottle feeding is to be condemned in its entirety because it is associated with high infant morbidity and mortality, especially in developing countries. Other hazards of bottle feeding include:-

a. Protein-energy malnutrition due to the problem of hygienic preparation of the artificial feeds by mothers.

b. Keratomalacia – resulting from low level of vitamin A in cow's milk.

c. Neonatal tetany – due to low level of calcium and magnesium in the bottle fed infant because these minerals are poorly absorbed from cow milk feeds.

d. Hypertonic dehydration: is a dehydration in which there is anorexia and irritability and sometimes convulsion with subsequent brain damage.

e. Obesity: Babies on artificial feeding on average, grow faster than breast-fed babies but are likely to become obese. This form of obesity may be the seed of future obesity.

f. Sudden infant death: A situation where an apparently healthy baby is found dead the next morning without any obvious cause. This sudden infant death or cot-death is more common in bottle-fed infants. Allergy to cow's milk has been suggested as a possible contributing factor in this most tragic situation. Recent studies also point to the position of the baby during sleep as contributory factor; prone position is less prone to sudden infant death than supine positions.

WEANING DIET: The time of weaning a child is of grave danger to him. After a fairly good supply of protein from breast milk, the quality of the diet drops suddenly to an extremely low and insufficient level by introducing predominantly starchy foods. Even when beans are added, the food is often too bulky for the small child to digest properly. However, if beans could be fed to the child as ground flour (beans soup), its utilization and subsequent assimilation would be improved remarkably. Weaning is the process whereby feeding from the breast is replaced partially or completely by the use of solid family foods.

Weaning should be done gradually over at least two weeks. Too sudden change of feeds can have disastrous consequences for the baby. During the process, solid foods are introduced one at a time, in minute quantities and at increasingly shorter intervals. Breast milk feeding should be withdrawn gradually by increasing intervals of breast feed and at the same time decreasing duration of sucking. The practice of waking up one day and painting the breasts with bitter leaves or quinine to prevent the child from sucking is psychologically traumatic and may leave permanent emotional defects in the child.

As mentioned above, infant formulas are not recommended for weaning because they could lead to childhood obesity due to their pleasant additives and high energy concentration.

Infant formulas, like all other manufactured foods, are high salt foods which when introduced to the child early in life could lead to hypertension in adulthood.

The pleasant taste of artificial formula foods may give an infant the "sweet tooth" which could eventually lead to excessive consumption of sugar predisposing him or her to dental caries and obesity.

The best weaning diet in our environment is red guineacorn/millet pap with Brewer's yeast, eggs, fish, vegetables, banana and avocado pear. Maize gruel should be avoided because of its low iron content, poor protein (zein) and nicotinic acid content.

CHILDHOOD NUTRITION

During childhood, the emphasis should be on providing the growing child with an adequate diet necessary for optimum growth. The child will require adequate amount of protein, carbohydrate, fat, minerals, fibre and vitamins. The major problem with childhood nutrition in the tropics is the severe shortage of protein in their diet. Growing children must be given high protein diet such as beans, fish, meat and eggs every day. Dairy products may also be given every day for optimum growth of the child depending on blood group compatibility. The dairy products must necessarily be of low-fat variety to prevent planting in the child the seed of future atherosclerosis, hypertension and heart disease. In this regard, the best product which has low-fat content and is good for children is dried, low-fat, skimmed milk.

The practice of denying children meat and eggs for the unfounded fear that they may become thieves later in life is to say the least very primitive and unacceptable. Such practice must be condemned. Children must be given top priority when it comes to meat and eggs because they need these foods for growth. Adults do not grow and therefore do not require much meat or eggs. In fact, these foods may prove detrimental to the health of adults in the long term in view of their high protein, cholesterol and saturated fat content.

I must hasten to add here, that it is unhealthy to over-feed children especially with junk foods. Overfed children may look plumpy and nice but they carry the seed of future obesity and its attendant complications. Research has shown that children who are obese early in life are more likely to grow up to be obese adults.

Children should be encouraged to eat unprocessed natural foods so that when they grow up they will stick to this healthy attitude of eating right for life-long vitality.

The key principle in childhood nutrition, therefore, is to make deliberate effort to provide high quality first-class protein foods in the family menu every day. The other aspects of nutrition like starch carbohydrates and fats usually take care of themselves. The pivotal role of every parent, therefore, is to see that at least one of the following food items is provided on the family dining table every day: beans, soyabeans, meat, fish, eggs, bambara nuts (okpa), milk and cheese. One other aspect of childhood nutrition that is woefully neglected in our society is fresh fruits and vegetables. Children need these foods for optimum growth.

The following fruits and vegetables are very good and should be provided daily at the dining table for all-round family health. They include: guava, orange, pawpaw, mangoes, pineapples, carrots, spinach, lettuce and cabbage. At least one of them must be consumed daily for the health of children.

However, for most children, a good mixture of vegetable proteins provides excellent growth in children. The best vegetable protein is in rice and beans. Eggs, lean meat and fish may be added to the mixture to further improve protein quality.

Vitamin requirements are relatively high in childhood which makes children more liable than adults to getting deficiency diseases. Since most Nigerian families cannot afford diets that supply all the vitamins needed for childhood growth, it is strongly advised that all children be given proprietary nutrients. The nutrients that are very crucial in childhood nutrition are summarized in the mnemonic: FIZCCAD, F = folic acid, I = iron, Z = zinc, C = calcium, C = vitamin C, A=vitamin A and D=vitamin D. These nutrients are crucial for children between the ages 6 months and 2 years. After this period, the growth usually slows down enough for vitamin needs to be met from adequate family food.

Vitamins A and D are best provided for the children from cod liver oil (Seven seas) given once or twice a week. Daily requirements of vitamin C can be gotten from citrus fruits and NUTRI-C, while folic acid is best taken in form of folic acid tablets daily. Zinc and iron are best supplemented in the form of zinc and iron tablets and from meat.

I strongly suggest that this practice be legislated for all parents to provide supplemental vitamins and minerals to children as their fundamental human right.

In conclusion, because our diet in the country is generally poor, we should focus attention on meeting the protein, mineral and vitamin needs of children. In order words, the major responsibility of all parents, therefore, is to ensure that beans, eggs, fruits, brown rice and vegetables are provided at the family table daily. In addition, proprietary cod liver oil, vitamin C and multi-minerals/multi-vitamins should be provided for all the family to satisfy the vitamin requirements of the entire family.

ADOLESCENT NUTRITION

Because of growth "spurt" of adolescence, these children require even higher amount of proteins than in early childhood. They also require supplements of vitamin C, A and D as well as iodine. Vitamins A and D as well as iodine are conveniently provided for by taking cod liver oil one tablespoonful once a week. Adolescent girls may require, in addition, supplemental iron twice a week and folic acid preparations daily because of menstrual losses. Their diet should also be adequate in starch, grains and tubers to spare available protein for optimum growth and energy which is highly needed at this active period of life.

NUTRITION IN THE ELDERLY

For a number of reasons, adults generally do not eat properly. The reasons include: lack of time, affordability, forgetfulness and unavailability of fresh foods, poor appetite, edentalousness and many more. These reasons make it imperative for elderly persons to take supplementary vitamins and mineral preparations on a regular basis for life-long health and vitality.

The vitamins that are easily missed in elderly nutrition include vitamins C, the B complex group and vitamin E. These vitamins along with vitamin A incidentally are crucial for the health of elders. This is because they act to reduce the rate of bodily wear and tear resulting from daily activities. In fact, vitamins A and C are said to slow down the ageing process as a result of their anti-oxidant activity by neutralizing harmful free radicals in the body.

For ease of dosing, it is better to take these vitamins separately rather than in one multi-vitamin tablet or pill. It is also advised that an elderly person take some vitamin C tablets daily as well as 3 tablespoonfuls of Brewer's yeast for all round health and vitality. The latter may be taken daily with breakfast. A rich source of vitamin E in our environment is sweet potato. This is a wonderful food indeed because its vitamin E content has been shown to significantly reduce the rate of the development of dementia in the elderly. Sweet potato is best taken boiled in its skin and eaten at breakfast (TABS). Another very good source of vitamin E is wheat, wheat-germ and wheat-germ oil. Wheat can be eaten boiled like rice or as whole-wheat brown-bread. Wheat is also rich in vitamin B complex, fibre and vitamin F. As emphasized elsewhere, wheat consumption should be strictly in accordance with blood group compatibility.

Other very important nutrients for our senior citizens include the sulphur-containing amino acids: methionine and cystine. They are thought to protect the liver and prolong life. The richest source of methionine in our environment is bambara nuts. This should be eaten regularly for life-long vitality. Bambara nuts can be eaten boiled and garnished with beniseed or ground into powder and cooked in the form of okpa. But okpa prepared in polythene bags is unwholesome and should be avoided.

Elderly people are particularly prone to constipation and other lower gastrointestinal tract diseases because their diet is often deficient in fibre. Beans are an all-round fibre food that is highly recommended for senior citizens. For life-long vitality therefore, elderly people should eat beans virtually every day. The beans could be eaten boiled, made into moi-moi or beans soup.

> The elderly should eat bambara nuts, avocado pear, sweetpotato, wheat, and beans regularly for life-long vitality.

The elders, for emphasis should eat all foods in moderation. A major objective of adult nutrition is avoidance of middle-age central obesity and its sequelae. Consumption of saturated fats should be reduced seriously and monosaturated fats should be used more liberally routinely. Smoking should be avoided completely. Alcohol may be consumed in small quantities, if at all.

Energy: Because of reduced physical activity, their energy requirements are correspondingly reduced from the average of 11.5MJ/day to about 8.5 MJ/day (~25%). The diet providing this reduced energy input is unlikely to provide all the necessary vitamins and minerals. Moreover, for various reasons, elderly people eat poorly. As mentioned above, reasons include among others: poor financial standing, poor appetite, and loneliness but it is better for the elderly to be underweight than overweight. They should eat calorie-restricted diet, by avoiding high calorie foods like powdered starch foods (amala, alibo, fufu and garri).

Protein: The amount of protein needed is just enough to meet the physiological need of bodily maintenance that is about 50g/day. The mixture of beans and brown rice will provide adequate protein. Addition of generous helpings of fish and egg regularly will be more than suffice.

Iron: Iron deficiency is common in the elderly, especially those on analgesic treatment for arthritis. Before they are put on iron supplementation, however, blood test should be done first to determine the type of anaemia for correct and holistic treatment.

Calcium: Calcium is necessary for regular heartbeat, normal muscle contraction and tone and nervous calmness and serenity. The calcium needs can be met through regular eating of calcium rich foods sources like baobab leaves, okra, locust beans, millet and green leaves.

As mentioned above, people are at very high risk of developing deficiencies of vitamin C and Vitamin B complex. A good supply of green vegetables is required to meet the need for folic acid and milk, liver, eggs and meat provide the other B vitamins. Where this is not practicable as in most families in the country, supplements of vitamins C and B complex could make all the difference between prolonged useful life and an early grave. A most pragmatic arrangement is to supply the old man or woman regular supplies of cod liver oil, Brewer's yeast powder, and vitamin C tablets instead of bottles of hot drink.

Finally, the elderly should avoid eating sugar and sugary foods including white sugar and pastries.

CHAPTER 29
GOOD NUTRITION ON A "SHOESTRING" BUDGET

"Scientific nutrition is the pillar of a longer, healthier and happier life"
(Gaylord Hauser)

Given that a "mudu" of rice now sells for between N350 and N500, a bottle of olive oil for N1,400 and the prices of other foodstuffs are similarly shooting up to the sky, it is almost impossible for an average citizen to provide an adequate diet for an average family at these "sappy" times.

Nevertheless, armed with the knowledge of the nutritional values of common foodstuffs as given in previous chapters, we are in a better position to shop for food items in such a way as to provide an adequate diet for an average family on a shoestring budget.

As mentioned elsewhere, the major goal of an adequate diet is to provide most of the essential nutrients daily. It should provide carbohydrate, protein, fat, vitamins, minerals and fibre in correct quantity and quality in one meal or at most within 24 hours.

Planning for an adequate diet therefore should begin before going to the market where we go to purchase the various food items. For most families who depend on monthly salaries, the planning should start before pay day so that most items may be purchased in bulk to save cost.

From dietary surveys across the country, the most grievous fault with our diet nationwide is the near absence of protective foods such as fruits and vegetables. The best way to ensure regular supply of fruits and vegetables daily is to open an account with a green grocer and pay in advance or in arears as the case may be. This way, one is sure to have fresh fruits and vegetables on one's dining table every day. As mentioned elsewhere, the best vegetables to eat are those in season.

After taking care of these protective foods, the next goal is to provide for high quality protein in our diet. As mentioned earlier the best source of protein for life-long vitality is a combination of plant protein, although we still require a little animal protein (eggs, fish and dairy products) to provide us with particular essential nutrients not readily present in plant protein sources.

The recommended plant proteins for life-long health include beans, soya beans, groundnut, lentils, and bambara nuts. Beans, especially, should be eaten daily in one form or the other for overall health. Good nutrition planning therefore requires that one purchase enough beans and bambara nuts at the beginning of the month to last for the month.

Purchasing about ten "mudus" of beans and five "mudus" of bambara nuts will provide enough plant source of protein for an average family of six per month.

In order to improve the biological value of plant proteins and to also provide some essential nutrients not readily found in plant proteins, one should eat some animal proteins like liver, eggs, cheese and fish, chicken or lean meat depending on blood group.

The most important aspect of starch carbohydrate is that when eaten fresh (boiled yam, sweet potatoes, and cocoyam) they provide fewer calories per gram compared to their processed forms like amala, garri, alibo or cereals. This calorie-restricted diet helps prevent middle-age obesity. Garri, alibo, amala, fufu and cereals are very high in calories and can easily lead to middle age obesity leading to premature death.

For good health, we should eat only healthy fats and oils. These healthy oils include the following: olive oil, soya oil, coconut oil, avocado oil, flaxseed oil, atili oil.

For soup making, the recommended ingredients include: Egusi, baobab leaves, locust beans (dadawa), beniseeds, bitter leaf, water leaf, spinach, beans, okra and green leaves – again, always choose according to blood group compatibility.

At the beginning of the month, an average family will do well to purchase and store up about 3mudu of egusi, 3 mudu of beniseed and 3 mudu of dry baobab powder.

The major point to bear in mind is that eating a diet low in saturated fats but rich in starchcarbohydrate along with fruits and vegetables has been shown to protect against cancer and heart disease.

Plant foods are low in Vitamins A, B_1, B_2 and B_{12},therefore, one should eat some animal protein daily as they contain these vitamins. The safest sources of animal protein for adults include: fish, chicken, eggs, fresh milk, cheese, turkey and bushmeat. Any other animal protein should be avoided, especially, pork, beef (farmed), mutton, pasteurized milk, powdered milk and goat meat.

Below is a table of the recommended food items and their current prices. One should be able to choose from the list according to blood group, taste and financial buoyancy without compromising on the principle of an adequate diet.

MONTHLY MEAL PLANNER FOR AN AVERAGE FAMILY OF SIX EARNING N400, 000 MONTHLY

S/N	FOOD ITEM 1	QUANTITY 2	UNIT COST 3 N	AMOUNT 4 N	% Food Expenditure 5	REMARK 6
1	Fruits/Vegetables	N/A	1000	30,000	22.2	Not negotiable
PROTEINS						
1	Beans	10 mudu	300	3,000	2.2	Not negotiable
2	Bambara nuts	2 mudu	400	800	0.6	
ANIMAL PROTEINS						
1	Fish			30,000	22.2	Not negotiable
2	Chicken	4 birds	2,000	8,000	5.9	
3	Bushmeat	3 kilos	3,000	9,000	6.6	
4	Crayfish	2 mudu	1,500	3,000	2.2	
5	Eggs	6 crates	750	4,500	3.3	
6	Skimmed Milk	1 large tin	1,500	1,500	1.1	
STARCH CARBOHYDRATE (CHOOSE ONE OR TWO ACCORDING TO TASTE AND BLOOD GROUP)						
1	Cocoyam					Breakfast
2	Sweet Potatoes			3,000	2.2	Breakfast
3	Irish Potatoes					Breakfast
4	Yams			6,000	4.4	Breakfast/lunch
CEREALS						
1	Acha					
2	Rice(Brown/Local)	20 mudu	350	7,000	5.2	Good for hypertension
3	Wheat					Good for elderly
4	Red	20	100	2000	1.5	For weaning

	Guineacorn	mudu				
5	Millet	10 mudu	100	1,000	0.7	For kunu

FATS AND OILS

1	Palm oil	1 gallon	1,500	1,500	1.1	Use sparingly if at all
2	Olive oil	1 gallon				Use ad Libertum Excellent
3	Coconut oil	2 bottles	1,500	3,000	2.2	Daily must
4	Sunflower oil	1 gallon				
5	Soyabean oil	1 gallon	4,500	4,500	3.3	

SOUP INGREDIENTS (CHOOSE DADAWA AND TWO OTHERS)

1	Egusi	4 mudu	750	3,000	2.2	
2	Beniseed	4 mudu	350	1,400	1.0	Appetizer
3	Boabab leaves	4 mudu	300	1,200	0.9	Excellent for children
4	Dadawa		1,000	1,000	0.7	The daily recommended
5	Redsweet pepper		1,000	1,000	0.7	Seasoning agent
6	Green leaves, Sweet green pepper & Tomatoes		3,000	3,000	2.2	Good for pregnant women
7	Seasalt		300	300	0.2	Seasoning agent
8	Onions		2,000	2,000	1.5	Appetizer

TREE NUTS (CHOOSE ONE OR TWO)

	Cashew nuts,		1,800	7,200	5.3	

	Almonds, Walnuts,				
TOTAL MONTHLY FOOD BUDGET			135, 400	100%	

From the table above, and for optimum health, a family should set aside at least 30% of their monthly income for food. From this amount, the given percentages for each food item should apply as calculated in column 5 of the table.

For example, take a family earning N50, 000 monthly

30% of this will be $\dfrac{30}{100} \times 50{,}000$

$= N15{,}000$

That means, N15, 000 should be spent on food. Out of this amount, 22.5% should be spent on fruits and vegetables.

$$\dfrac{22.5}{100} \times 15{,}000$$

$$= N\,3{,}375$$

25% of N15, 000 is N3, 375.

Using the table, you can calculate your food budget based on your monthly income.

For good planning, therefore, an average family of six should purchase the following animal proteins at the beginning of every month in accordance with their financial capabilities: dressed chickens, bushmeat, ice-fish, crates of eggs and a large tin of skimmed powdered milk. Fish, especially, should be eaten at least 2-3 times a week. The caution with fish is the potential for mercury poisoning, one should avoid large fish and fish from polluted water. The fibre content of our diet is grossly inadequate. In planning an adequate diet, one should first and foremost try to correct this most serious flaw by providing fruits, vegetables and legumes on our dining tables every day. There are two possible ways of achieving this: one is to set aside a calculated amount of money that will cover the whole month. The only problem here is the high chance of misappropriating the money so set aside. A better way of achieving this noble goal is to buy fruits and vegetables twice a weekby handing over the total money to your grocer to deduct from it as you buy weekly.

CHAPTER 30
FOOD AND KITCHEN HYGIENE

"The higher the quality of food, the better; and for health, never rely upon the delicacy of cooking"
(Confucius, 2000 BC)

Food, if not properly handled can quite easily be a source of all kinds of diseases–the so-called food-borne diseases. Examples of diseases that can easily be transmitted through food include:

1. Typhoid fever8. Trichiniasis (emulates 50 different diseases)
2. Tuberculosis   9. Salmonellosis
3. Brucellosis   10. Streptococcal infection
4. Poliomyelitis   11. Staphylococcal food poisoning
5. Coxsackie viruses   12. Ascariasis
6. Amoebic dysentery
7. Tapeworm

As can be seen above, the list of diseases that can be contracted from eating unhygienic or contaminated food is quite long. It is almost a miracle that people do not fall ill more often. The notion that Africans brought up in unhygienic environments are immune to these diseases is highly fallacious. The high morbidity and mortality rates in our society attest to the falsity of this claim.

So how can one prevent this long list of diseases from marring one's life? There are several approaches:

1. At the communal level: health education, legislation and enforcement of sanctions to ensure proper disposal of human waste as well as the treatment of potable water by government will go a long way to control most of these diseases.

2. The heating of left over foods in the morning before eating is the single most important factor why people who live in unhealthy environments do not fall ill every day. This is so because most disease-causing bacteria are easily destroyed by minimum heating.

3. At the home base, preventive nutrition requires that all those who prepare the family food must wash hands frequently using soap. They must wash hands every time they enter the kitchen and more so after they visit the toilet. All left-over foods must be covered and before they are consumed again, they must be heated up, even if they have been stored in the refrigerator because cold does not kill bacteria but only prevents their

multiplication. So that, whenever the food is thawed the bacteria begins to grow again.

4.	To keep disease carrying animals at bay, the kitchen must be kept squeaky clean always. All bits of food must be cleaned out because they tend to attract animals like cockroaches. And if possible, kitchen doors and windows should be protected with fly-proof screens. To rid the kitchen and the whole house of cockroaches, spray the corners of the kitchen and rooms with black pepper. And each door should have half door attached.

5.	Household pets like cats and dogs must not be allowed near the kitchen, because their faeces can transmit diseases to man.

6.	If you go to a restaurant, and you find the person handling food to have sore throat, catarrh, or any skin disease, it is best to politely walk out of such a restaurant to avoid contracting food poisoning.

g.	To prevent bacteria from producing poisonous toxins in cooked food, the food must be cooled rapidly after cooking (put in cold water). If food is allowed to stand and cool down slowly, it provides bacteria with optimum conditions to elaborate toxic poisons into the food. The bacteria survive cooking in the form of "spores" and can easily go back to their active form when conditions are right e.g. when food is allowed to cool down slowly over a long time. Rapid cooling of cooked food prevents spores from reverting to their active forms.

Still on the kitchen, the best way of washing up utensils after meals is to use hot water with powdered detergent and the plates left to dry in air. The practice of wiping plates with towels after washing up is not recommended because the towels may introduce harmful bacteria unless they are washed after every meal.

On the issue of utensils, it is better to use glass cups and plates throughout and avoid plastic utensils because their use is linked to certain forms of cancers as they tend to leak harmful chemicals into drinks and foods. And worst of all, plastic containers must never be used for storing drinking water because it has been shown that plastics dissolve into water to cause cancer. Similarly, it is best to purchase cooking oils in metal containers than plastic bottles or worse, polythene bag.

With regards to cooking pots, only steel and cast-iron cooking pots maybe used for cooking food. Cast iron pots have been known to impart a small amount of elemental iron to cooked food which prevents iron deficiency anaemia in family members that share food from such pots. On the other hand, aluminum pots are not to be used at all because they can cause serious illness on long term use. Moreover, cheap aluminum pots, the type used for group cooking at ceremony like weddings, commercial cooking at "Bukka", restaurant and schools (see picture) is loaded with poisonous heavy metal. It is therefore much better to spend more money on iron or steel pots than to buy cheap aluminium pots that will cause illness to family members in the long run. Traditional African clay pots are safe and should be used inplace of aluminium pots.

Finally, the practice of cooking moi-moi and okpa wrapped in polythene bags must be strongly condemned across the country because the polythene bag is potentially very harmful.

So also, the practice of wrapping kosai, suya or raw akamu in newspapers is to be seriously discouraged because the papers impart a significant amount of poisonous lead metal directly into the food so wrapped.

CHAPTER 31
FOOD AND SEXUAL HEALTH

"The foundation of perpetual youth is good nutrition"

(Garylord Hauser)

Sexual health is of such importance to the African and especially the Nigerian male that a book on preventive nutrition would be considered incomplete without pointing out what to eat and what not to eat in order to preserve sexuality right into old age.

For the general preservation of the sex organs, first class proteins such as bushmeat, fish, eggs, turkey and chicken are invaluable. They work best when complemented with foods that are rich in vitamin B complex (Brewer's yeast) and vitamin E in wheatgerm or wheatgerm oil daily.

From time immemorial, through trial and error, certain foods have been found to promote sexuality; these are termed aphrodisiacs. They tend to stimulate sexual desire and improve performance. Other foods have been found to decrease sexual desire and performance. These are referred to as anaphrodisiacs or anti-aphrodisiacs.

Aphrodisiacs

Many plant foods, especially those that create flatulence promote erection. The Latin Poet Martial (d. AD 104) once said that "if your wife is old and your members languid these vegetables and legumes can do more than fill your belly". These include beans, peas and lentils. Others that help promote and maintain sexual health from day to day include: garlic, onions, radish, carrots, spinach, pepper, dates (dabino), thyme, rice, wheat and ginger (TABS and TAMS).

Seafoods are popular aphrodisiacs because of their very high zinc and phosphoric content. They include cod fish, trout, and eggs of fish (cod roe), crayfish, crabs, shrimps, prawns, periwinkles and snails.

Some insects are thought to be great aphrodisiacs, especially the winged variety. A good example is "shinge" or white termites that are harvested during the early rainy season in Northern Nigeria. Research work from Zaria has shown that termites have very high level of phosphorus (4th richest) and iron. It is also the richest source of riboflavin and 3rd richest source of niacin in our environment.

Honey, particularly the unprocessed, is said to be a superlative sex invigorator, especially, if mixed with alligator pepper.

The flesh of some reptiles like snakes is popular aphrodisiacs in oriental countries. Animal flesh in general is said to be aphrodisiac, especially brain, liver, testicles and lean meat.

Milk and milk products like cheese are also excellent. Onions soups with fish (the popular Nigerian fresh fish pepper soup) is said to be infallible as an aphrodisiac.

Alcohol in all its forms has strong aphrodisiac properties but only if taken in very small quantity. Any large quantity would give the desire but kill the act.

I must take this opportunity to warn all readers of this book that some substances may be very powerful aphrodisiacs but can destroy the sex organs after some time. They have even killed many a hypertensive patient because of their strong stimulating effect on the central nervous system. They should therefore never be used! These powerful but harmful aphrodisiacs include: nightshade (belladona), nux vomica (strychnine), throng apple (datura), cannabis, hashish, yohimbine, bamboo shoots (China), ginseng (from China), and quebracho (from South America).

Cantharidum from Africa is often mistaken for "spinach" and may cause family epidemic of mental confusion, restlessness and signs of atropinization. Treatment is with 5-10 mg neostigmine ½ hourly till patient recovers.

The Anaphrodisiac foods: As mentioned above, these foods depress sexual desire and kill erection. They include: nutmeg, cabbage, lettuce, cucumber, dried coriander, coffee and tea in excess, lemon, orange, vinegar, soda water, sweets (which contain menthol) soft drinks and grape fruits.

Tobacco and snuff, although strictly-speaking are not foods, yet they are patronized by a lot of ignorant people and therefore deserve special mention here. Tobacco and snuff are serious anaphrodisiacs. Indeed it has been said that there is a latent antagonism in the male body between tobacco and women, so that a taste of one diminishes the taste and capacity for the other. For this reason, most people who want to maintain their sexual health must eschew smoking. A famous physician once said "any man who smokes cigars, and drinks soda water can sleep with my wife"; so sure was he that such a man would be impotent. A recent study in London, England, has shown that most smokers (75%) have serious problems with sexual potency.

Apart from food, one's lifestyle can also affect one's sexual potency. Silk clothing enfeebles the erectile powers of the sex organs by engendering bodily warmth.

Indeed, most modern man-made fabrics are harmful for the same reason. There is no substitute for cotton and woolen clothing for preserving one's sexual health. One must insist on white 100% cotton underwear all the time.

With respect to ambient temperature both cold and heat are harmful. Cold inhibits successful performance. Too much warmth, especially around the genitals is detrimental. So also detrimental is the tight constriction of the organs with pants. Tight pants reduce potency. The same applies to sitting for long periods in a chair or a car e.g. office workers and long distance drivers. Horse riding is especially detrimental. Hippocrates (d. 359 BC) wrote that the Scythians (who were great horse riders) had great difficulty in erecting as a result of long periods spent on the saddle. Consequently, the Scythian race died out.

Any excess of eating, drinking, sleeping, hard physical labour or exercise can also depress sexual urge and performance. One exception is walking which is done at a moderate pace. Walking is supposed to have a wonderful effect on the vitalic nerve plexus at the crotch whereas sitting in one place interferes with the nerve plexus. Anyone wishing to reduce his sexual potency should avoid walking. I personally walk briskly for 30 minutes every other morning and the result is a blissful marital life.

Finally, worry, fear and anxiety all actively inhibit desire. So does too much brainwork, especially mathematics, which is highly detrimental to the amorous instinct. According to Benjamin Walker, a prostitute once told the world renowned mathematician, J.J. Rousseau (d. 1778) "to leave women alone and study mathematics".

ERECTILE DYSFUNCTION (ED)

As erectile dysfunction (ED) is related to variety of health concerns, it is important that a man who is struggling with sexual performance should go for thorough physical medical examination to discern the root cause for proper treatment. The following supplements are useful in ED.

1. Viagra – only works in 2/3 of men who use it. It also causes a variety of undesirable side effects including hearing loss
2. Flaxseed oil
3. Arginine – check liver and kidney functions before placing a patient on it.
4. Gingko biloba – better than viagra
5. Zinc – does not fail

6.   Vitamin E – wheat-germ oil + Evening Primrose Oil
7.   Vitamin C heightens intensity of orgasm
8.   DHEA
9.   Bioflavonoids
10.   Acupuncture

SUMMARY OF FOODS THAT AFFECT SEXUAL POTENCY

S/N	APHRODISIACS	ANAPHRODISIACS
A	**Protein**	
	Bushmeat; Milk Powder; Cheese, Eggs, Offal, Fish, Snake, Chicken, Turkey, Beans, Shinge, Peas, Snails, Snail Powder, Crayfish, Crabs, Periwinkle, Shrimps, Red Meat	Soya products, Lentils, Hard Cheese, Chickpeas
B	**Supplements**	
	Brewer's yeast, Pumpkin seeds, Jobelyn, Sesame seeds	MSG
C	**Minerals**	
	Kelp, Zinc, Magnesium, Sea salt	
D	**Cabohydrates**	
	Honey, Brown Rice, Wheat	
E	**Amino acid supplements**	
	Arginine, Histidine, Glutamic Acid	
F	**Vegetables**	
	Radish, Onions, Garlic, Ginseng, Sweet Red Pepper, Sweet Green Pepper, Carrots, Broad Leafed Spinach, Ginger	Cabbage, Small Leafed Spinach
G	**Fruits**	
	Pinapple, Figs, Avocado Pear, Dates	
H	**Oils/fats**	
	Olive Oil,Avocado Oil, Wheatgerm Oil,Evening Primrose Oil, Coconut Oli	Groundnut Oil, Palm Oil, Palm Kernel Oil

A careful observation of the above will show that most of the items listed under aphrodisiacs are listed in TABS and TAMS. What a glorious combination!

CHAPTER 32
WHAT THEN SHALL WE EAT?

"For good health, one should eat that which one would rather not eat and avoid that which one would rather eat".

(Anonymous)

While preparing this book, someone put it to me like this: "doctors always say we should not eat this or that; this food causes cancer; the other causes ulcer and another causes goiter; what exactly do you want us to eat then?" I was not at all surprised at the question because, many people had put the same question to me over and over again and I intend to answer this most important question in this chapter.

First and foremost, the essence of this book is to raise awareness about the nutritional value or potential hazards of common foods found in our environment. If the awareness influences our general attitude towards healthy eating, my job would have been done.

The major objective of the book therefore is to sensitize people on the need to stick to native and homegrown foods and to avoid harmful, junk and alien foods as much as possible. The best food is said to be that which is grown or cultivated in one's own locality; and for each season, the fruits and vegetables of that season are best.

In order to avoid making an already complicated subject more complicated, I will summarize what I would tag the life-long super nutrition programme by simply listing the different foods under their functional classifications.

Carbohydrates: The safe carbohydrates include:

(1). Starchy root crops: yams, cocoyams, sweet potatoes and Irish potatoes. They are low in energy content and are good for slimmers and those who want to maintain their body weight into ripe old age.

(2). Cereals: The following cereals are safe and are produced in the country. They include: brown rice, wheat, guineacorn, acha, millet.

Protein: The animal sources of protein include: fish, eggs, bushmeat, chicken and turkey. Beef, mutton and goat meat should only rarely be eaten because of their saturated fat content. Pork is best avoided. Offals should be eaten once a week for their vitamin B complex content as well as iron.

Fats: The best oil to use on a regular basis isolive oil and coconut oil. Palm oil may be used only sparingly as when needed for preparing traditional soup such as "egusi" or "alapa" soups. Vegetable oils like soyabean oil whch are manufactured by solvent extraction in hydrocarbon solvents may not be entirely safe because contaminants from the process can cause cancer. It is better to use vegetable oils that are obtained through cold-compression method e.g. Extra-virgin olive oil.

Cholesterol and Health

Ancel Keys, who studied cholesterol extensively in the fifties said categorically: cholesterol in food (including eggs) does not have any impact on cholesterol in the blood. The more correct cause of high blood cholesterol is refined carbohydrates (sugar) in manufactured foods. The other cause is genetic predisposition leading to the different types hyperlipidaemias.

Fruits and Vegetables: Most vegetables grown in the country are safe and good for health. The only precaution is that they should be washed properly and where possible cooked before eating because of the unhygenic way they are produced. Cabbage should not, however, be consumed too often because of the high level of goitrogens it contains. Spinach with small foliage is not recommended for regular consumption because of the same reason. Popular vegetable soups are good provided they are not over cooked.

Vegetables are best consumed blended or juiced, and to aid the absorption of Vitamin A, D, E and K, always add natural Fulani butter, olive oil or avocado oil.

Vitamins: several dietary surveys have confirmed that the vitamins that are notoriously deficient in typical African diets include vitamin A, B_2,and C. Vitamin A intake is best improved by green vegetables and yellow fruits. Where this is not possible or where there is exaggerated physiological need such as in the first year of life, pregnancy and lactation, supplementation through cod liver oil 2 times a week may be appropriate. The administration of vitamin A to infants as part of the national programme of immunization is a laudable effort.

Vitamin B_2 has been tagged the "longevity vitamin" because it has been shown to prolong life by 10% in laboratory animals. Its requirements, however, is difficult to meet through eating commonly available foods. The daily requirements of this and other rare vitamins like pantothenic acid, inositol, biotin, choline, and para-aminobenzoic acid (PABA), are best met by consuming Brewer's yeast daily and taking liver once a week.

Vitamin C requirements are also difficult to meet in the African diet because it is not stored in the body and must be taken daily. In addition, our traditional cooking methods destroy virtually all the vitamin C available in fresh foods (except in sweet potatoes). Since fruits are not very popular, if one must take in Vitamin C daily, supplementation with proprietary vitamin C is appropriate. Indeed, in view of its large margin of safety, coupled with its vital role in the body, vitamin C is one of the few vitamins recommended for daily consumption to complement dietary supply. I personally take 500mg twice a day for all round health daily. Vitamin C improves the absorption of iron and calcium, hence the addition for daily supplementation of this very important vitamin.

Minerals: The three minerals that are notoriously lacking in the African diet are calcium, iron and zinc. Although the body can easily adapt to low calcium levels in the body, it is best to meet the suggested daily requirements of calcium of about 500 – 800 mg. This is especially true for growing children, pregnant women and lactating mothers. The increased requirement is best met by eating non-dairy products like fish bones, baobab leaves (miyan kuka), green leaves, locust beans (dadawa), sesame seeds and mazankwaila. Mazankwaila is a very practical means of meeting bodily calcium needs, especially, for growing children where it can be used as a sweetener for the whole family. It also supplies enough iron to meet daily requirements of this vital element for growing children. An indirect intake of calcium is through cod liver oil, because the latter contains Vitamin D that improves calcium absorption from the intestines. In order to avoid Vitamin D toxicity from cod liver oil, it is best to take it just once a week. This is because vitamin D is stored in the body and does not have to be taken on a daily basis.

Iron requirements are extraordinarily increased for growing children. Iron needs are best met through eating meat, liver and eggs. A very pragmatic source would be mazankwaila if this is used as a sweetener on the family dining table. Iron needs for pregnant women can also be met through eating meat and mazankwaila but more often than not, supplemental iron is needed as well. Iron needs of the whole family can also be met by using cast iron pots used for cooking rather than aluminium pots.

Fibre: The World Health Organisation (WHO) recommends that for good health, a person should consume at least 30g of fibre every day. High fibre foods are thought to protect against the development of certain diseases of the colon like cancer, diverticulitis, and hemorrhoids. A high fibre diet is also beneficial in that is slows down the rate of glucose and fat absorption from the small intestine, thus reducing the chances of developing Type 2 diabetes and arterial disease. The causes of both diseases are related to the rate of rise in blood glucose (glucotoxicity) and fat concentrations respectively in the absorptive periods after eating.

The best local sources of fibre include fruits, vegetables, cereals and legumes such as beans. Vegetable soups, which are popular in Nigeria, are highly recommended for daily consumption. Fruits are available year round and those in season are best. The fibre in beans is particularly desirable as it has been shown to lower blood cholesterol. It also helps reduce body weight and lowers blood sugar levels in diabetics.

CHAPTER 33
"DAILY MUSTS" FOR HEALTH

"The longer I live, the less confidence I have in drugs and the greater is my confidence in the regulation and administration of diet and regimen"

(John Redman Coxe)

Bearing in mind that about 100 million cells are replaced daily in our body, one can only imagine the immensity of chemical reactions that go on every millisecond in the body; tearing down senescent cells and building up new ones all at the same time. The degree of dynamism is mind boggling and all must get it right first time in order to prevent diseases or worse, death. Given the enormity of the activities taking place every second and every minute, the body will require to have in place the right type of building materials at all times in the form of nutrients to obtain the best end result of rebuilding the body.

The science of nutrition has been able to show that for the body to carry out its rebuilding activities successfully and optimally, the body needs to have access to a complement of 91 nutrients. Very few food items come close to having all these 91 nutrients in them. The one that readily comes to mind is bee pollen which is tagged the "world's perfect food". Some food items do not have all the 91 nutrients but contribute hard-to-find nutrients and are therefore, called "superfoods". Combining two or three superfoods brings one close to attaining the ideal requirement of 91 nutrients.

Superfoods have high concentration of hard-to-find nutrients and are therefore tagged DAILY MUSTS for health. They can be combined in meals (TABS and TAMS) to attain near perfect complement of nutrients. They include things like Brewer's yeast, honey and cereal sprouts (tsiro).

Some nutrients are easily destroyed by heating or cooking, therefore, their source must be consumed raw. The raw foods containing these heat-sensitive nutrients are also considered superfoods. In addition, some nutrients are not stored in the human body for more than 24 hours and therefore their food sources must be eaten daily for optimum health. These nutrients include vitamin C, the mineral zinc and vitamin B_2. Their food sources of these nutrients are also labeled superfoods because they contribute to health and longevity of a person.

In summary, below is a table of some of the foods and supplements that should be selected from daily if one is to maintain health into ripe old age. They are the foods that I have tagged "Daily-Musts" for Health.

S/N	NAME
1	Green tea
2	Cinnamon
3	Coconut oil
4	*Gingko biloba*
5	Sweddish bitters
6	Cocoa powder
7	Carrot
8	Avocado pear
9	Moringa
10	Sesame seeds
11	Apple cider vinegar
12	Flaxseed oil
13	Red wine
14	Soy milk
15	Beetroot juice
16	Onions
17	Garlic
18	Tomato sauce
19	Walnuts
20	Almonds
21	Eggs
22	Soya beans
23	Brown rice
24	Brewer's yeast
25	Sardines
26	Salmon
27	Lemon juice
28	Watermelon
29	Fish
30	Apples
31	Pomegranate
32	Copper containers (for drinking water)

33	Royal jelly
34	Evening primrose
35	Cayenne pepper
36	Grape seed extract
37	Probiotics
38	Dates
39	Tree nuts (Brazil, Walnut, Cashew, Almonds)
40	Coconut powder (rich in zinc for ED)
41	Grape juice (red)
42	Mango
43	Guava
44	Kiwi
45	Broccoli
46	Cabbage
47	Sunflower oil
48	Cauliflower
49	Spinach
50	Lettuce
51	Sweet potatoes
52	Tomatoes
53	Pawpaw
54	Chocolate bar
55	Milk thistle
56	Turmeric
57	Lecithin
58	CoQ10
59	Oleander extract
60	Vitamin D_3 caps/injection
61	Wheatgerm oil
62	Yoghurt
63	Spirulina
64	Cordyceps
65	Betaine HCL for all elderly 50 and above
66	Chitosan

67	Kola nut
68	Propolis plus capsules
69	Bitter kola
70	Ginger
71	Gotu cola
72	Aloe vera
73	Kelp
74	Zinc lactate
75	Vitamin E
76	Olive oil (Extra virgin)
77	Bambara nuts
78	Psyllium powder
79	Cod liver oil essential (7-alive) Combo
80	Parsley
81	Sea salt (Brittany)
82	Beans
83	Molasses (not processed)
84	Tiger nuts
85	Multivitamin/multi mineral (Reload)
86	Calcium pantothenate
87	Honey
88	Mustard seed powder
89	Pancreatic enzyme (those above 45 years)
90	Vitamin B_{12} (for those above 40 years)
91	Nutmeg
92	L – Glutamine
93	L- Arginine
94	L- Carnitine
95	L- Carnosine
96	Dr. Affi's Mracle – Shake
97	Dr. Affi's Breakfast Salad

CHAPTER 34
SUPREME IMPORTANCE OF BRAIN HEALTH
"Your brain, the seat of life"
(Friedrich Nietzsche)

It is the brain and not the heart or liver that is the seat of life and soul. The brain, therefore, is our most precious asset that must be protected and nourished and nurtured to last as long as possible.

No matter how fit the other parts of your body may be, if the brain is not functioning optimally, the rest of the body will become ill and diseased sooner than later. On the other hand, if the brain is functioning optimally, then the rest of the body will also function correctly and the whole body will become healthy.

Indeed, scientific evidence has shown that if the brain is supported nutritionally to produce the entire complement of pituitary, pineal and hypothalamic hormones in their right quantities and quality all year round, life expectancy can be extended almost indefinitely. This is because all other parts of the body are connected to and controlled by the brain. It is therefore extremely important for us to know how to eat correctly and do other things necessary for us to preserve and promote the health of the most precious asset that we have. In fact, if properly done, optimum nutrition can enable our bodies get healthier even as we get older chronologically. For example, I personally feel healthier and happier now at 59 years than I have ever felt all my life. In other words, I am getting healthier as I get older chronologically.

The story of Daniel and his friends as recorded in the Bible, has more than adequately established that a simple change of diet can improve brain health and performance by a factor of ten (10) and within ten (10) days simply by adopting a non-flesh diet rich in fruits and vegetables. And still another biblical example, Caleb at 85 years old was as strong as he was at the age of forty.

Age, they say, is a thing of the past. Agelessness can be our double portion and within our reach if only we can make appropriate changes in our lifestyles and diet to ensure the optimal functioning of our brains.The good news is that you can take steps to keep your memory sharp at any age. And still another Biblical example is the story of Caleb who was 85years but was as strong as a 40years old person.

The following lifestyle and dietary changes will do just that:

1.   Aerobic Exercise

Exercising in fresh, open air is one of the best ways to keep your brain fit and functional right unto ripe old age. Exercise improves cognitive function by a factor of 10 – 15%, which is quite phenomenal considering that man at present is utilizing only 5% of his brain capacity. During exercise, there's increased development of capillary circulation with increased blood supply boosting nutrients and oxygen supply to the brain cells. Some researchers have been able to show that exercise actually causes enlargement of the brain area concerned with memory: specifically, the caudate lobe.

Just 30 minutes of brisk walking or gentle jogging (roving) in fresh air 5 times a week will do the magic.

2. Sleep

An adult person needs 7 to 8 hours of sleep to maintain optimum cognitive function. Seven hours of sleep is already too small. The earlier one gets to bed, the better. In addition, one needs 20 minutes of siesta daily to further sharpen the brain.

3. Brain Foods

Eating the right foods according to blood group and avoiding harmful foods will increase mental performance by a factor of 10, leading to mind boggling and far reaching positive consequences for health. And this can be achieved within 10 days if done properly. Remember Daniel in the Bible. The fundamental principle is to ensure that one eats in accordance with one's blood group and avoid all those items that are harmful.

The next important principle is to eat in such a way that the body is supplied with all the 91 nutrients that are necessary for optimum health and longevity within 24 hours.

The acquisition of these 91 nutrients for perpetual health can be achieved as follows:

- **Eat coloured (rainbow) fruits and vegetables**. They are excellent for brain health. Examples include: broccoli, avocado, cabbage, walnuts, onions, garlic, green leaves cauliflower and blueberries.
- **Fish and Fish Oil:** eating oily fish 50g per week is excellent for brain health. Examples include: salmon, herring, sardines, mackerel and tuna. Pregnant women who ate just 50g per week of the above listed fish gave birth to children with significantly higher IQ scores and lower risk of behavioural problems and fewer difficulties with fine motor skills,

communication and social development. Where fish is difficult to come by, mercury-free Seven Seas cod liver oil 10ml once a week will do quite well.

- **Soya oil:** Taking just one teaspoonful at bed time improves brain function dramatically.

- **Green Tea**: Drinking two cups of green tea, in addition to other health benefits, is thought to improve memory and prevent age-related memory loss(dementia)

- **Cocoa Powder:** Taking cocoa powder in just very small quantity ($^1/_2$ tsp) daily improves mental function with specific reference to spatial arithmetic and mathematics.

- **Eggs:** Taking at least one egg (organic) daily improves brain function, helping brain development in children and memory recall in adults.

- **Restricted Calorie Diet:** Eating sparingly improves memory and cognitive function. This is achieved by avoiding foods of high glycaemic load (GL). These high GL foods include powdered grains and powdered root/tuber starch such as amala, alibo, semovita, acha, garri – the so-called "swallow" in Nigeria. This is so because the process of drying root starch and the processing of grains into powder increases their calorie content by 300% thereby, rendering them very unhealthy for regular consumption. Boiled   starchy root carbohydrates have low glycaemic load. They include: boiled yam, cocoyam and sweet potatoes.

- **Wheat-germ and Wheat-germ oil:** Taking wheat-germ and wheat-germ oil daily improves cognitive brain function by above 45%. This is attributed to the high vitamin E present in wheat-germ. Moreover, wheat-germ is very rich in the mineral zinc which is very important for optimal brain function. Wheat-germ and wheat-germ oil are devoid of harmful gluten, so blood group O persons can take them without any problem.

- **Coconut Oil:** As mentioned under cooking oils, coconut oil is the veritable brain health booster per excellence. Taking coconut oil (one tablespoon) daily will boost brain function and prevent or even treat Alzheimer's disease.

- **Adequate water drinking:** Adequate water drinking 1.5litres early in the morning and every two hours by the clock is vital for top–rank performance of the brain. Even a slight dehydration of 2% (which may be imperceptible to the person) could lead to 10% decrease in brain function and this is a profound loss, especially in the ability to take decisions. This happens long before the thirst sensation sets in. The thirst sensation sets in only when dehydration has approached 3% body weight and by then a lot of damage has already been done.

- **Lecithin:** This is the most important brain food available and needs to be taken as a supplement in liquid form or as granules. A very small amount (2 teaspoonfuls) daily is all that is needed to do the job. It contains inositol and choline for grey hair treatment as well as for optimum brain function. In addition, lecithin is excellent for heart health as well as in helping obese people lose weight. It takes 4 – 6 weeks to seethe full effect of taking lecithin. Lecithin is also referred to as the "Patron Saint" of the body because of its extreme importance to health and longevity.

- **Rosemary:** Rosemary flower is superb for brain health.

- **Beniseed:** It is very rich in lecithin and polyunsaturated oil that is excellent for brain function especially, for students. Taking one handful of fresh raw beniseed is all that is needed daily.

- **Tomatoes:** Eating cooked or fresh tomatoes boosts intellectual performance because of its rich content of glutamic acid that is very essential in the metabolism of glucose–the only source of energy for the brain. Therefore taking tomato soup at breakfast prepared for both children and adults is essential for optimal functioning of the brain throughout the day.

- **Gotu-Kola:** This is also known as "memory herb". It stimulates brain function, especially creative function and learning ability. It also reduces mental fatigue and forgetfulness. As a result of its effect on the brain, it secondarily elevates sexual drive and improves sexual performance.

- **Ginseng:** Ginseng improves memory and strengthens appetite. It is said to boost stamina and support sexual energy. The activity of ginseng is greatly improved when taken along with gotu-kola, ginger, green tea,   cayenne pepper andcinnamon.

- **Alcohol:** In small amount–1-2 drinks per week–decreases the risk of cognitive decline.

- **Apples:** Eating fresh apple at night (red apple is best) protects the brain against free radical damage. Apples contain quercetin that protects brain cells from radical damage. Eat apples peeled. Taking ½ an apple at bedtime is all that is required.

- **Grape seed Extract:** Taking supplements of grape seed extracts daily prevents cognitive decline into ripe old age.

- **Kola Nuts:** Although kola nut has caffeine, the caffeine is natural without additives. Kolanut has been shown to improve long term memory, protect the heart and prolong life. I normally take one kola nut early before my morning work out to help with weight loss and protect against arrhythmias and heart attack during exercise.

- **Olive Oil:** Taking 2tablespoonfuls of olive oil daily either directly or as salad dressing will boost cognitive function through elevation of serotonin levels in the brain. Olive oil or atili oil should be the main cooking oil in the house which could be supplemented with coconut oil, avocado oil, soya oil (at night) cod liver oil and wheatgerm oil.

> The six (6) brain oils include; olive oil, avocado oil, flaxseed oil, codliver oil, wheatgerm oil and soya oil

- **Pituitary Stimulators:** This group of foods works directly to stimulate the pituitary gland and hypothalamus for perpetual youthfulness and agelessness. According to some authorities, "By just taking care of the hypothalamus and the pituitary glands, you can virtually live forever". The pituitary stimulators include:

S/N		S/N	
1	Bee Pollen	10	Royal Jelly (Quartely)
2	Soya bean products (genistein)	11	Sesame Seeds (1 handful daily)
3	Evening Primrose oil	12	Walnuts (3 times a week)
4	Zinc	13	Yam (arginine) regularly
5	Manganese	14	Watermelon (arginine) seeds
6	Turmeric	15	Wheagerm and wheatgem oil (vitamin E)

7	Ginseng (Red Korean)	16	Snail Powder (L-Glutamine)
8	Sunflower Seed	17	Coconut oil and coconut powder
9	Vitamin B_{12} injection 100 mcg monthly	18	Liver once a week (preferably at weekends)

Minerals and Health

Scientists have been able to demonstrate that mineral elements in the diet are necessary for you to remember, think and feel emotions. They include: boron, copper, iron and manganese.

S/N	Mineral	Food Sources
1	Boron	Apples – at bedtime (peeled)
2	Copper	Kelp, Dulce, Fresh Vegetables and Fruits
3	Iron	Red Meat and Liver
4	Zinc	Organ Meats, Ginger, Wheatgerm and Coconut powder
5	Manganese	Pineapple, Millet and Quaker Oats

Fats and Brain Health

It takes just 24 days (less than one month) for the fat in the diet to alter the physical composition of the brain. So it is important to bear this all important point in mind to ensure you consume only fats and oils that are healthy.

Generally speaking, saturated fats (diary fats, palm oil, palm kernel oil and meat) decrease one's ability to think and remember things while polyunsaturated fats (soya bean oil, olive oil and sunflower seed oil) help you think.

Breakfast

For proper and perpetual brain health the most important meal to eat is a good and heavy breakfast that is rich in high quality protein, healthy oils and complex carbohydrates that have low glycaemic index and low glycaemic load (boiled sweet potatoes, boiled yam, boiled cocoyam and brown rice). Taking Dr. Affi's Breakfast Salad brings you up close to an ideal breakfast for a super-performing brain on a daily basis.

Multivitamins and multi-mineral food supplements: Regular taking of multivitamins and multi-mineral food supplements for top-gear performance of the brain daily.

Yoga: Especially asana headstand and shoulder stand.

Green leaves: Especially green cabbage contains phosphatidylserine (PS) that improves memory and concentraton.

Red wine: Especially the type made with Pirot Noir grapes has the highest concentration of resveratrol that boosts brain function. It is particularly good for blood group O persons.

High ORAC foods: Like prunes, raisins and sorghum bicolor (Jobelyn)are great brain health boosters. They can literarily reverse the hand of the aging clock. (ORAC means OxygenRadial Absorbance Capacity).

S/N	Food Supplements	ORAC
1	Sorghum Bicolor	37,000
2	Prunes	5,770
3	Raisins	2,500

- **Almonds/Walnuts:** Almonds and walnuts are very rich in copper for grey hair. They also improve memory. This is particularly true for walnuts because the nut with its convoluted surface resembles the surface of the human brain.

CHAPTER 35
IDEAL BODY WEIGHT

"Your body is the baggage you must carry through life; the more excess the baggage, the shorter the trip you are likely to take"

(Anonymous)

The size of a person's body has a direct influence on his or her health and longevity. For a given age, height and body frame, there is an ideal body weight that makes for optimum health and vitality.

Being overweight predisposes one to certain diseases like diabetes mellitus, hypertension, gallbladder stones and heart disease. On the other hand, if a person is underweight, he or she is predisposed to diseases such as peptic ulcer, psychiatric disorders, endocrine disorders as well as unexplained early death.

A number of parameters have been used to determine whether or not one is within an acceptable size for one's age, height and frame. These include straight weight taking, chest measurement and so on. These measurements, although alright for research, are not good enough for general use.

Recently, a new measurement that proved versatile and satisfactory has been introduced into clinical practice. This measurement is called the body mass index (BMI). It is the ratio of a person's weight in kilograms divided by the square of his height in metres as follows:

$$\text{Body Mass Index (BMI)} = \text{Weight (kg)} \div \text{Height (m)}^2$$

The usefulness of the body mass index is based on the fact that a person's weight is related to the square of his height in metres. The ratio is easy to calculate and is also widely accepted. Research work has been able to show that a person's health and longevity is directly related to his or her body mass index as shown below.

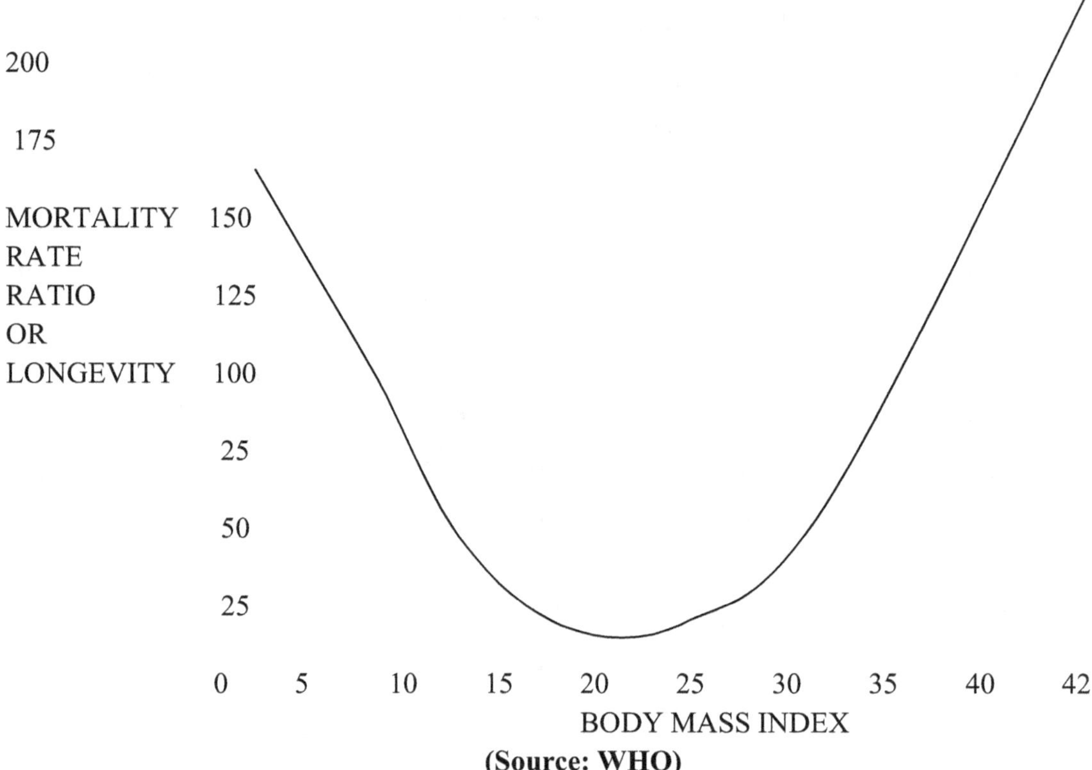

(Source: WHO)

The figure above shows that BMI range between 18.5 and 24.9 is associated with lowest percentage mortality ratio. Outside this range, the mortality rises on both sides but more sharply on the right (over-weight) side. For optimum health and vitality therefore, it is important that one maintains his or her weight at a level that gives a BMI of between 18.5 – 24.9.

One can calculate the range of desirable body weight for any given height using the formula:

$$BMI = \frac{Wt.kg}{Height\ (m)^2}$$

For a man who is 1.63 metres (5ft. 4 inches) the range of desirable body weight is therefore as follows:

For Lower Limit (BMI =18.5)

$$BMI = \frac{Weight\ (kg)}{Height\ (m)^2}$$

That is, Weight (kg) = BMI x Height (m)^2

$$= 18.5 \times 1.63^2$$
$$= 18.5 \times 2.66$$

$$= 49.2 \text{ kg}$$

For upper limit weight (BMI = 24.9)

$$= 24.9 \times 1.63^2$$
$$= 24.9 \times 2.66$$
$$= 66.2 \text{ kg}$$

So the desirable range of weight for a person of height 1.63m is within 49.2 – 66.2kg (range interval of 17kg).

Since the range of desirable weight for each individual height is so wide, it is expedient to introduce the concept of body frame to take into consideration the varying skeletal make up of persons with the same height, in order to have a more precise ideal body weight. For convenience as well as convention, human adults are divided into three categories of body frames: small, medium, and large. There are several measurements that help in this categorization but the simplest approach is the use of ankle circumference. The measurement is taken just above the two prominences present on each side of the ankle joint. If one's ankle circumference is less than 21cm (8inches), the person is said to be of a small frame. Between 21 – 23 cm (8''- 9") the person is of medium frame and above 23cm one is said to have a large body frame. With the help of the above measurements one can determine his or her own exact desirable body weight from the following tables of normals.

TABLE I: DESIRABLE WEIGHT (kg) FOR MEN 25 YEARS AND OVER

Height (Metre)	Small Frame ankle circumference <21 cm	Medium Frame ankle circumference 21 – 23 cm	Large Frame ankle circumference > 23cm
1.57	50.4 – 54.0	53.1 – 58.0	56.7 – 63.5
1.60	51.8 – 55.4	54.4 – 65.9	58.0 – 64.8
1.63	53.1 – 56.7	55.8 – 61.2	59.4 – 66.6
1.65	54.5 – 58.1	57.2 – 62.6	60.7 – 68.7
1.68	55.8 – 59.9	58.5 – 64.4	62.1 – 68.2
1.70	57.6 – 61.7	60.3 – 66.2	63.9 – 72.5
1.73	59.4 – 63.5	62.1 – 68.4	66.2 – 75.0
1.75	61.2 – 65.3	63.9 – 70.2	68.0 – 76.5
1.78	63.0 – 67.5	65.7 – 72.0	69.8 – 78.3
1.80	64.8 – 69.3	65.7 – 74.3	71.6 – 80.55

1.83	66.6 – 71.7	69.3 – 76.5	73.8 – 82.8
1.85	68.4 – 72.9	71.1 – 78.8	75.6 – 85.0
1.88	70.2 – 75.2	72.9 – 81.0	77.9 – 87.3
1.90	72.0 – 77.0	75.2 – 83.3	80.1 – 90.0
1.93	73.8 – 87.8	77.4 – 85.5	81.9 – 91.8

TABLE II: DESIRABLE WEIGHTS (kg) FOR WOMEN AGED 25 YEARS AND OVER

Height (Metre)	Small Frame	Medium Frame	Large Frame
1.47	41.4 – 44.1	43.2 – 48.15	46.8 – 53.6
1.50	42.3 – 45.5	44.1 – 49.5	47.7 – 54.9
1.52	43.2 – 46.8	45.5 – 50.9	49.0 – 56.3
1.55	44.6 – 48.2	46.8 – 52.2	50.4 – 57.6
1.57	45.9 – 49.5	48.2 – 53.6	51.8 – 59.0
1.60	47.3 – 50.9	49.5 – 54.9	53.1 – 60.3
1.63	48.6 – 52.2	50.9 – 56.7	54.5 – 62.1
1.65	50.0 – 53.6	52.2 – 58.5	56.3 – 63.9
1.68	51.3 – 55.4	54.0 – 60.8	58.1 – 65.7
1.70	53.1 – 57.2	55.8 – 62.6	59.9 – 67.5
1.73	54.9 – 59.0	57.6 – 64.4	61.7 – 69.3
1.75	56.7 – 60.8	59.4 – 66.2	63.5 – 71.1
1.78	58.5 – 63	61.2 – 68.0	65.3 – 72.4
1.80	60.3 – 64.8	63.0 – 69.8	67.1 – 73.1
1.83	62.1 – 66.6	64.8 – 71.6	68.9 – 77.9

For women between 18 – 25 years of age subtract 0.45kg for each year under 25.
A simple but less accurate method of determining one's acceptable body weight is to read off the maximum and minimum weight based on the calculated maximum and minimum body frame factor. See table below.

TABLE III: DESIRABLE RANGE OF BODY WEIGHT FOR PERSONS AGED 25 YEARS OVER

Height (Metre)	Minimum Desirable	Maximum Desirable

	Weight (BMI = 18.5)	Weight (BMI = 24.9)
1.57	45.6	61.4
1.60	47.4	63.7
1.63	49.2	66.2
1.65	50.4	67.8
1.68	52.2	70.3
1.70	53.5	72.0
1.73	55.4	74.5
1.75	56.7	76.3
1.78	58.6	78.9
1.80	59.9	80.7
1.83	62.0	83.4
1.85	63.3	85.2
1.88	65.4	88.0
1.90	66.8	89.9
1.93	68.9	92.8

In conclusion the body mass index is a useful and easily determined ratio that serves to remind us to keep within desirable range of body weights compatible with longevity and long-life day-to-day vitality.

To maintain a desirable body weight, the diet prescribed in this book will go a long way to make this possible. However, for permanent long-term achievement and maintenance of an ideal body weight, one needs in addition to the prescribed diet in this book, a sustained and regular programme of moderate physical exercise. I intend to deal more fully on this very important topic of exercise for vitality in a separate book.

CHAPTER 36
24 HR RITUAL FOR 24/7 VITALITY

"When it comes to eating right and exercising, there is no 'I'll start tomorrow'.......tomorrow is a disease"

Terri Guillemets

After having spent over 10,000 hours reading books and reviewing scientific journals on nutrition over the last 30 years, I have been able to come up with a simple time-table of rituals that would enable health seeking persons put into practice the dietary and other non-food activities necessary to keep one healthy and vibrant 24 hours each day.

As a pragmatist who likes to reduce complex problems into simple activities that most people can follow, I have tried to reduce the bewiffering information on food and nutrition to simple steps without losing the essentials. I have set out to reduce the complex innumerable foods into groups that can be consumed in 24hours while at the same time, providing the all nutrients that can lead to perpetual youthfulness and longevity.

The diet advocated is just a guide which people can adapt to suit their unique dispensation and events of the day.

On waking up at 4.30am, I begin with morning with prayers for one hour. Thereafter, I break my overnight fast by drinking 1 litre of bottled water – part of the daily water therapy. Following that, I take 1 tablespoonful of raw unheated honey, 1 tablespoonful of olive oil and then I follow it up with my soaked 'combo' (2 dates, and 1 handful of black sesame soaked overnight in a copper bowl). The last thing I eat before I set out for my morning workout is half a white kolanut. With this early morning ritual, I am now set for the morning work-out. I leave the house by 5.45am and head for the field to join my faithful exercise colleagues at 6.00am to work out for one hour. By 7.00am, we all disperse. On getting back home, I drink another 250ml of bottled water to make up for the dehydration from sweating on the field.

Next, I engage in the following exercises while listening to BBC World Service:

    a. Push-ups – 50

    b. Pull-ups – 10

    c. Squatting – 25

    d. Woodcutters weight lifting – 10

    e. Neck exercises – 5

    f. Eye exercises – 5

This group of exercises takes till 7.30am, the time for family devotion which takes 15minutes. Next I go for breakfast which takes 20minutes and follows the given strict order:

a. Protein – egg (boiled), fish, beans or meat (according to blood group)
b. Fruit – watermelon, pineapple, mangoes
c. TABS (See Appendix)

Then lastly, you wash down the breakfast with a cup of green tea. To bring up the best from the green tea (anti-oxidants, catechins, polyphenol), it is necessary to add the following: lemon juice, cinnamon, apple cider vinegar, ginger (fresh or powder), cayenne pepper and pomegranate juice.

You would have noticed that from 5.00am when I woke up, I never mentioned teeth brushing until after breakfast. This is to ensure that the food particles are properly brushed away after eating breakfast. The brushing is postponed till after bathroom rituals like shaving and emptying the bowel before you come to brush. This is to prevent the brushing away of the soft enamel of teeth caused by food just eaten.

Once you are through from the bathroom, you proceed to prepare and go to work. For the rest of the day while at work, you continue to drink water at odd hours of the clock starting with 250ml of bottled water at 9.00am. Thereafter, you wait till 11.00am to drink 500ml of bottled water. Lunch time is between 1.00pm to 2.00pm. The lunch should ideally be starchy root carbohydrates (boiled/pounded yam, roasted yam, boiled sweet potatoes, cocoyam, and Irish potatoes).

Thomas Affi's Miracle Shake

This is a fully-raw mixture of daily must items listed at the appendix. This could be taken as a stand-alone lunch or it may be taken before the swallow mentioned above.

The TAMS is touted to reverse aging by removing wrinkles of age to give a person natural face lift. Your eyes become bright and clear as evidence of bodily detoxification. Hair becomes thicker and grey hair darkens. One becomes slimmer (belly-busted). It also improves brain function leading to clear thinking, memory improvement and emotional equanimity. The TAMS literally makes a person become 10x smarter and wiser than one was a few weeks before.

After the TAMS, taken between 12noon to 12.15pm, one is allowed to drink 250ml of water after 30minutes. If one still wishes to take lunch, it can be taken after about 30 minutes after drinking the water. One could also take as snack any fruit in season if he or she so wishes (mangoes, guava, cashew).

At around 5pm, one is expected to take another 250ml of water in anticipation of dinner/supper at 6.30pm – 7.30pm. Before dinner, one should do 50 press-ups or weight lifting and do yoga. The dinner should be decidedly light and mainly uncooked food with one or two eggs (boiled) to promote sound sleep. Mainstay items for dinner include: brown rice Quaker oats, bambara nuts Tiger nuts sweet potatoes and fruits (watermelon, pineapple, and avocado). The dinner should be washed down with a hot cup of herbal tea (chamomile) along with one teaspoonful of raw honey, ¼ tsp of cinnamon; 1 teaspoonful of soya oil or olive oil, one date and a pinch of turmeric.

The dinner or supper time should not exceed 7.30pm so that one could pass urine before bed at 9 – 10pm before retiring. Ideally, when properly done, one should sleep soundly from 10.00pm to 5.00am without any interruptions to pass urine in the night. This is nature's way that a normal person does not wake up to pass any urine at night. Any change in this normality should signal dietary indiscretion or disease. Accordingly, appropriate steps should be taken promptly to elucidate the cause and remedy it early.

The final ritual before bed is to take one's time (at least 5 minutes) to brush the teeth thoroughly to remove any food bits that may remain to cause dental decay or mouth odour in the morning. After brushing the final ritual is to evacuate the rectum and followed by the body wash for peaceful night rest.

In summary, in drawing up the above rituals I have taken into consideration virtually all the important principles for a correct diet appropriate exercise five days a week but resting 48hours (on Saturdays and Sundays) to allow the body recuperate. For maximum effect, I have included one day fast on Saturdays for spiritual and physical upliftment.

All the food items captured are at the right quantity, the right quality and are taken at the right time and sequence for effective optimization of health. You just need two to three months of trial of this diet and its rituals to change your life forever!

Remember also, that throughout the 24 hour ritual, there's no place for deep frying of food items in the family kitchen. Even cooked food is at a minimum. The focus is to consume high quality animal protein (10%), fruits and vegetables (400g), starchy-root boiled carbohydrates (70% energy), and healthy oils (20%).

The TABS is 80% raw food and the TAMS, almost 90% raw food. This level of achievement has brought us close to the ideal of fully-raw food diet which is believed to be the secret or the holy grail of perpetual youthfulness and longevity.

CHAPTER 37
CAVEAT EMPTOR

"Extremism in healthy eating can become an illness called orthorexia nervosa"
(Anonymous)

Knowledge of good nutrition and correct choice of food can be extremely rewarding if carried out in moderation.

However, some people take the concept to extreme, where their mental and physical health is compromised often without them knowing it. The condition where this extreme behavior is allowed to affect the health of the person is referred to as orthorexia nervosa. The patients are usually well educated middle class persons in their 30's. These people tend to fixate on quantity rather than quality of food. They rigorously eliminate sugar, salt, coffee, alcohol, wheat, gluten, yeast, soya beans and maize from their diet. They religiously avoid any food they believe is tainted with pesticides, herbicides or hormones (so-called non-organic foods). An exception is the avoidance of foods that are selected based on allergy and/or blood group incompatibility.

This extreme practice of avoiding an entire group of foods can leave the victims malnourished. In addition, such imposed rigidity in the choice of food can put a strain in relationships, particularly, family and friends. So that as we teach and read about correct choice of food for healthy living, it is important to bear in mind the wisdom of moderation in everything. For instance, it is believed that if one can score 80% in the correct choice of food, one is doing very well, already. One doesn't have to become neurotic about it as long as one observes the basic scientific principles underlying the choice of foods. It would be most unwise to lay down any specific rules about what precise foods people should eat or not eat for health. This is so because environment, personal idiosyncrasies, culture and economy have to be taken into account when prescribing a diet for a particular group of people. For instance, the Eskimos cannot be expected to live on the same food as the Masai people of Kenya. Nevertheless, no matter where one lives, some general principles of quantity, quality, timing and combinations apply across the board since we have the same flesh, blood and body systems.

This book is coming at a time when the emphasis in medicine practice and health worldwide is changing drastically from hospital-based curative, to community-based preventive approach. The focus is now on self-control and primary prevention of disease rather than on the expensive hospital-based management of disease conditions which have hitherto proved unaffordable and often unsafe in some cases.

APPENDIX A

BLOOD GROUP A

BENEFICIAL FOODS	NEUTRAL FOODS	FOODS TO AVOID COMPLETELY
MEATS None	**MEATS** Chicken, Turkey, Guinea fowl, Ostrich.	**MEATS** Beef, Buffalo, Goose, Heart, Lamb, Liver, mutton, Partridge, Pheasant, Pork, Rabbit, Veal, Bushmeat, Duck, Squirrel.
SEAFOODS Carp, Cod, Mackerel, Salmon (fresh), Trout, Sardine, Snail, Perch(silver, yellow), White Fish, Pollack, Red Snapper, Monkfish.	**SEAFOODS** Swordfish, Sturgeon, Tuna, Shark, yellowtail, Tilapia, Trout(brook), Sailfish.	**SEAFOODS** Anchovy, Bluefish, Catfish, Caviar, Crab, Crayfish, Eel, Frog, Haddock, Lobster, Flounder, Sole, Herring, Shrimp.
BEANS Adzuki, Black-eyedPeas,Green beans, Red beans, Soya cheese' Lentils, Pinto, Black beans, Broad beans.	**BEANS** Green Peas, White Beans, Jicama, Mung-beans/ Sprout.	**BEANS** Chickpea, Kidney, Lima, Navy, Tamarind, Copper beans.
EGGS/ DAIRY Soya milk.	**EGGS/ DAIRY** Goatmilk, Mozzarella, Goatcheese, Egg (chicken, duck, quail, Goose), Yoghurt.	**EGGS / DAIRY** American cheese, Cottage cheese, Milk (all) Parmesan, Butter, Butter milk, Cheddar, Cream cheese, Gouda, Ice-cream.
NUTS / SEEDS Flaxseed, Pumpkin seeds, Groundnut, Groundnut butter, Walnuts.	**NUTS/ SEEDS** Almond, Chestnut, Sesameseed, Sunflower, Sesame butter(Tahini).	**NUTS/ SEEDS** Brazil nuts, Cashew, Pistachio, Cashew butter.

OILS	OILS	OILS
Linseed, Olive, Walnut, Flaxseed	Cod liver, Canola, Atili, Soy, Sunflower, Sesame, Wheatgerm, Safflower, Evening PrImrose, Avocado	Maize, Castor, Cottonseed.
CEREALS	**CEREALS**	**CEREALS**
Amaranth, Oat bran, Buckwheat, Oatmeal.	Barley, Cornflakes, Rice, Maize, Millet, Rice bran, Maize, Semovita, Guineacorn, Spaghetti.	Wheat, Whole Wheat Bread products, Biscuits, White flour.
VEGETABLES	**VEGETABLES**	**VEGETABLES**
Alfalfa, Beet green, Broccoli, Carrot, Dandelion, Garlic, Horseradish, Leek, Okra, Onion, Parsley, Parsnips, Pumpkin, Kale, Ginger, Celery, Romaine lettuce, Spinach, Turnips.	Asparagus, Cucumber, cauliflower, Beet, Coriander, Maize (all), Kelp, Lettuce (Boston), Mushroom (Portobello), Radish, Shallot, Squash, Cocoyam, Watercress.	Cabbage (red/white), Yam, Chili pepper, Eggplant, Mushroom (Shiitake), Olive (black), Pepper (all), Tomato, Irish potato (all)

BENEFICIAL FOODS	**NEUTRAL FOODS**	**FOODS TO AVOID COMPLETELY**
FRUITS	**FRUITS**	**FRUITS**
Apricot, Blackberry, Plum, Blueberry, Cherry, Fig, Prune, Grapefruit, Lemon, Pineapple.	Apple, Red/Blackcurrant, Date, Elderberry, Goose berry, Grape, Guava, Kiwi, Lime, Melon, Peach, Pear, Pomegranate, Strawberry, Watermelon,	Banana, Coconut, Mango, Orange, Pawpaw, Plantain, Tangerine, Melon (bitter).

	Raisin.	
JUICES Carrot, Celery, Grapefruit, Pineapple, Aloe, Cherry, Lemon, Spinach, Blackberry, Apricot. Lime, Prune.	**JUICES** Apple, Apple cider, Cranberry, Cucumber, Grape, Vegetable (from acceptable vegetables), Cabbage, Guava, Pear.	**JUICES** Orange, Tomato, Coconut milk, Mango, Pawpaw.
SPICES/CONDIMENTS Barley malt, Blackstrap molasses, Garlic, Ginger, Mustard, Soy sauce, Turmeric.	**SPICES/CONDIMENTS** Allspice, Almond extract, Basil, Brown sugar, Chocolate, Kelp, Cinnamon, Coriander, Cumin, Curry, Dill, Dulse, Honey, Maple syrup, Nutmeg, Vanilla, Thyme, Oregano, Paprika, Peppermint, Rosemary, Sage, Saffron, Stevia, Cassava, Lecithin, Brewer's yeast .	**SPICES/CONDIMENTS** Ketchup, Mayonnaise, Pepper (all), Wintergreen, Acacia (gum Arabic), Pickles, Tamarind, Vinegar (all)
BEVERAGES Coffee, Green tea, Red wine, Water (alkaline).	**BEVERAGES** White wine	**BEVERAGES** Beer, Liquor, Minerals, Soda water.
HERBAL TEAS Alfalfa, Aloe, Chamomile, Fenugreek, Echinacea, Ginseng, Ginger, Milk Thistle, , Astralagus, Gentian, Rose Hip, Dandelion, Saint-John's wort, Valerian, *Gingko biloba*, Fennel.	**HERBAL TEAS** Chickweed, Dong quail, Peppermint, Sage, Hops, Skullcap, Thyme, Yarrow.	**HERBAL TEAS** Black tea, Cornsilk, Cayenne, Goldenseal, Catnip.

BLOOD GROUP B

BENEFICIAL FOODS	NEUTRAL FOODS	FOODS TO AVOID COMPLETELY
MEATS Lamb, Goat, Rabbit, Bush meat.	**MEATS** Beef, Buffalo, Liver (calf), Pheasant, Turkey, Veal, Ostrich.	**MEATS** Chicken, Duck, Goose, Squirrel, Heart, Partridge, Quail, Guinea Fowl, Pork.
SEA FOODS Mackerel, Sardine, Cod, Salmon (fresh), Shad, Perch (Ocean), Halibut, Haddock, Sturgeon, Sole (except Gray or Dover).	**SEAFOODS** Catfish, Herring (fresh), Rainbow, Swordfish, Tuna, Tilapia, Perch (White, Yellow or Silver)	**SEAFOODS** Crayfish, Frog, Snail, Shrimp, Crab, Oyster, Bass, Trout, Sole (Gray or Dover).
BEANS Lima, Kidney, Navy.	**BEANS** Broad, Copper, Green peas, Green beans, White.	**BEANS** Black-eyed peas, Chickpeas, Soya beans and Soya bean products, Black beans, Lentil, Mung beans/sprout, Adzuki.
EGGS / DAIRY Cottage cheese, Goat cheese, Milk (Cow or Goat), Yogurt (All), Ricotta, Mozzarella	**EGGS / DAIRY** Buttermilk, Cheddar Gouda, Egg (Chicken), Ghee.	**EGGS/ DAIRY** American cheese, Ice-cream, Blue cheese, String cheese, Egg (Duck/Goose/Quail).
NUTS/ SEEDS Walnut (Black)	**NUTS/ SEEDS** Almond, Flaxseed, Brazil nuts.	**NUTS/ SEEDS** Cashew, Groundnut, Groundnut butter, Pumpkin seed, Sesame seeds and butter, Sunflower.
OILS Olive, Atili.	**OILS** Cod liver, Flaxseed, Evening primrose,	**OILS** Avocado, Canola, Corn, Sunflower, Cottonseed,

	Wheatgerm, Walnut, and Almond.	Soya bean, Coconut, Groundnut, Safflower, Sesame, Castor.
CEREALS Millet, Oat bran, Oat meal, Rice, Brown Rice.	**CEREALS** Barley, Wheat bread, Quinoa.	**CEREALS** Maize, Cornflakes, Wheat, Rye, Couscous, Semovita, Noodles, Pasta, Spaghetti, Cassava, whole Wheat bread, Buckwheat, Wheat germ.
VEGETABLES Beet, Broccoli, Brussels sprout, Carrot, Cauliflower, Parsley, Mushroom (Shiitake), Eggplant, Kale, Parsnip, Mustard green, Sweet potato, Beet green, Ginger, Pepper (all), Yam (all),Cabbage (all).	**VEGETABLES** Celery, Cucumber, Radish, Dill, Garlic, Ginger, Lettuce, Leek, Mushroom (Common/Domestic), Okra, Onion, Irish Potato, Shallot, Scallion, Spinach, Squash, Turnip, Kelp, Seaweed, Watercress, Zucchini.	**VEGETABLES** Avocado, Maize, Black Olive, Pumpkin, Radish, Tomato, Artichoke, Rhubarb.

BENEFICIAL FOODS	**NEUTRAL FOODS**	**FOODS TO AVOID COMPLETELY**
FRUITS Banana, Cranberry, Grape, Plum, Watermelon, Pawpaw, Pineapple.	**FRUITS** Apple, Apricot, Plantain Blackberry, Blueberry, Cherries, Kiwi, Fig, Red/Blackcurrant, Date, Gooseberry, Elderberry, Grapefruit, Guava, Pear,	**FRUITS** Coconut, Pomegranate. Avocado, Bitter melon, Starfruit, Persimmon

	Lemon, Lime, Mango, Melon, Orange, Peach, Prune, Raisin, Raspberry, Strawberry, Tangerine.	
JUICES Cabbage, Beet green, Cranberry, Pawpaw, Pineapple.	**JUICES** Apple cider, Apple, Aloe, Lime, Apricot, Tangerine, Tomato, Cherry, Coconut milk, Carrot, Celery, Cucumber, Grapefruit, Orange, Lemon.	**JUICES** Coconut, Pomegranate, Tomato.
SPICES/CONDIMENTS Cayenne, Curry, Ginger, Horseradish, Parsley, Pepper.	**SPICES/CONDIMENTS** Basil, Caraway, Carob, Kelp, Chocolate, Coriander, Clove, Cumin, Dulse, Dill, Lecithin, Honey, Molasses, Thyme, Vanilla, Mustard, Nutmeg, Oregano, Paprika, Pepper, Vinegar, Turmeric, Bergamot, Garlic, Peppermint, Rosemary, Sage, Brewer's yeast.	**SPICES/CONDIMENTS** Stevia, Soy sauce, Acacia (Arabic gum), Corn syrup, Aspartame, Dextrose, Almond extract, MSG, Barley malt, Carrageenan, Pepper (black/white) Cinnamon. Cassava, Cornstarch, Gelatin (plain).
BEVERAGES Green Tea	**BEVERAGES** Black tea, Coffee, Red wine, White wine, Beer.	**BEVERAGES** Liquor (distilled), Soda (Diet/Cola/Club).
HERBAL TEAS Ginger, Ginseng, Licorice, Parsley, Peppermint, Raspberry leaf, Rose hip, Milk thistle, Cayenne, Green.	**HERBAL TEAS** Alfalfa, Thyme, Chamomile, Chickweed, Dandelion, Echinacea, St. John's wort, Fenugreek Sage, Astralagus,	**HERBAL TEAS** Aloe, Corn silk, Goldenseal, Hops, Red clover, Stinging nettle root, Skullcap, Shepherd's purse.

| | Valerian, Strawberry leaf. | |

BLOOD GROUP AB

BENEFICIAL FOODS	NEUTRAL FOODS	FOODS TO AVOID COMPLETELY
MEATS Turkey.	**MEATS** Lamb, Mutton, Rabbit, Liver, Pheasant, Ostrich, Goat.	**MEATS** Squab, Beef, Chicken, Duck, Goose, Heart, Partridge, Pork, Turtle, Horse, Squirrel, Quail, Guinea fowl, Bushmeat.
SEAFOODS Cod, Mackerel, Salmon (fresh), Sardine, Snail, Tuna, Sturgeon, Pickerel, Red Snapper, Pike.	**SEAFOODS** Bluefish, Catfish, Caviar, Carp, Herring (fresh), Shark, Swordfish, Perch, Tilapia, White fish.	**SEAFOODS** Crab, Crayfish, Eel, Frog, Salmon (Roe), Shrimp, Oyster, Halibut, Lobster, Trout (all), Sole (all).
BEANS Lentil, Navy, Pinto, Soya beans and Soya beans Product, Green beans.	**BEANS** Broad, Green Peas, Copper, Lentil (Domestic/Red), White, Tamarind.	**BEANS** Black, Kidney, Lima, Fava, Chick pea, Black-eyed peas, Adzuki, Mung beans/ Sprout.
EGGS / DAIRY Cottage cheese, Goat cheese, Farmer Cheese, Mozzarela, Milk (Goat), Protein shakes, Yogurt.	**EGGS / DAIRY** Eggs(Chicken/Goose/Quail), Cheddar, Cream/String cheese, Milk (Cow, Skim), Soya milk.	**EGGS / DAIRY** American cheese, Blue cheese, Ice-cream, Milk (Cow, Whole), Ice cream, Duck eggs, Butter.
NUTS/ SEEDS Chestnuts, Groundnut, Groundnut butter, Walnuts.	**NUTS / SEEDS** Almond, Brazil, Cashew, Macadamia, Flaxseed.	**NUTS/ SEEDS** Pumpkin, Sesame, Sunflower.
OILS Olive, Walnut.	**OILS** Almond, Wheat germ, Canola, Cod liver, Flaxseed,	**OILS** Safflower, Cottonseed, Sesame, Sunflower,

	Groundnut, Soya bean, Evening primrose.	Coconut.
CEREALS/ GRAINS Quaker oats, Brown Rice, Millet, Guinea corn, Rye, Amaranth.	**CEREALS/ GRAINS** Rice, Oats, Couscous, Wheat germ, Quinoa, Barley, Wheat-bran, Whole-wheat.	**CEREALS/ GRAINS** Maize, Cornflakes, Cassava.
VEGETABLES Alfalfa, Avocado (Florida), Beet, Collard, Beetgreen , Broccoli, Cauliflower, Celery, Cucumber, Dandelion, Eggplant, Kale, Mushroom (Maitake), Mustard green, Parsley, Parsnip, Sweet potato, Yam, Garlic.	**VEGETABLES** Spinach, Bamboo shoot, Cabbage, Carrot, Lettuce, Mushroom (Common/Domestic), Okra, Olive, Onion, Irish potato, Scallion, Shallot, Squash, Tomato, Turnip, Leek, Cocoyam, Watercress, Kelp, Ginger.	**VEGETABLES** Aloe, Avocado (California), Cauliflower, Maize, Olive (black), Radish, Mushroom (shiitake), Pepper (all), Pickle, Rhubarb.

BENEFICIAL FOODS	**NEUTRAL FOODS**	**FOODS TO AVOID COMPLETELY**
FRUITS Cherry, Cranberry, Fig, Gooseberry, Grapefruit, Grape, Kiwi, Pineapple, Lemon, Plum, Watermelon.	**FRUITS** Apple, Blueberry, Blackberry, Blackcurrant, Date, Lime, Melon, Pawpaw, Pear, Peach, Plantain, Prune, Raisin, Raspberry, Strawberry, Tangerine.	**FRUITS** Banana, Coconut, Guava, Mango, Orange, Pomegranate, Starfruit, Bitter melon, Avocado (California).
JUICES Cabbage, Carrot, Celery,	**JUICES** Apple cider, Apricot,	**JUICES** Guava, Mango, Orange.

Cranberry, Cherry, Lemon.	Blackberry, Apple, Cucumber, Tangerine, Grapefruit, Tomato, Pineapple, Pawpaw, Prune, Pear, Lime.	
SPICES/CONDIMENTS Curry, Garlic, Horseradish, Molasses, Parsley, Oregano, Ginger.	**SPICES/CONDIMENTS** Basil, Brown sugar, Dill, Chocolate, Clove, Dulse, Coriander, Cumin, Jelly, Ginger, Honey, Jam, Kelp, Maple syrup, Sage, Marjoram, Turmeric, Molasses, Mustard, Nutmeg, Peppermint, Rosemary, Cinnamon, Stevia, Thyme, Vanilla.	**SPICES/CONDIMENTS** Allspice, Almond, Cayenne, Corn starch, Ketchup, Pepper (all), Cassava, Vinegar (all), Aloe, MSG, Aspartame, Guar gum, Soya sauce, Dextrose, Maltodextrin, Sucanat, Fructose, Invert sugar, Barley-malt, Brewer's Yeast.
BEVERAGES Green Tea.	**BEVERAGES** Red wine, Club soda, Beer, White wine.	**BEVERAGES** Black tea, Coffee, Soda (Cola/Diet).
HERBAL TEAS Alfalfa, Chamomile, Echinacea Ginseng, Ginger, Rose hip, Strawberry leaf, Fenugreek, Astralagus, Parsley, Milk thistle.	**HERBAL TEAS** Dandelion, Sage, Peppermint, Thyme, Valerian, Chickweed, Saint-John's wort, Goldenseal.	**HERBAL TEAS** Aloe, Cayenne, Cornsilk, Gentian, Red clover, Senna, Skullcap, Hops, Rhubarb, Shepherd's purse.

BLOOD GROUP O

BENEFICIAL FOODS	NEUTRAL FOODS	FOODS TO AVOID COMPLETELY
MEATS Beef, Lamb, Liver, Heart, Bushmeat.	**MEATS** Chicken, Duck, Partridge, Goose, Pheasant, Guinea fowl, Ostrich, Rabbit, Turkey, Squirrel.	**MEATS** Pork, Quail, Turtle
SEAFOODS Cod, Swordfish, Red snapper, Perch, Halibut, Sole (except Gray or Dover), Tilefish, Bass, Trout, Shad, Sturgeon.	**SEAFOODS** Crayfish, Crab, Tuna, Sardine, Mackerel, Tilapia, Oyster, Herring (fresh), Snail, Shrimp, Salmon (fresh).	**SEAFOODS** Barracuda, Catfish, Salmon (roe), Octopus, Herring (Smoked/Prickled).
BEANS / LEGUMES Blacked–eyed pea, Adzuki.	**BEANS / LEGUMES** Black, Broad, Chickpea Green beans, Lima, Peas, Red beans, Soya beans.	**BEANS / LEGUMES** Copper, Kidney, Navy, Tamarind, Lentil.
EGGS/ DAIRY None	**EGGS / DAIRY** Egg (chicken/duck), Butter, Cheese, Goat cheese, Soya milk, Mozzarella.	**EGGS / DAIRY** Milk (cow & goat), Yoghurt (all), Cottage Cheese, Ice-Cream, Egg (Quail/Goose), Cheddar.
NUTS/ SEEDS Flaxseed, Pumpkin seed, Walnuts (Black/English).	**NUT S/ SEEDS** Almond, Almond butter, Macadamia, Sesame seed, Sesame butter (Tahini).	**NUT S/ SEEDS** Brazil nut, Cashew, Chestnut, Groundnut, Groundnut butter, Pistachio, Sunflower Seed/Butter.
OILS Linseeds, Olive, Flaxseed, Atili.	**OILS** Canola, Cod liver, Sesame, Almond, Walnut.	**OILS** Maize, Cotton seed, Groundnut, Coconut, Avocado, Evening primrose, Safflower, Soya

		bean, Castor.
CEREALS/ GRAINS None	**CEREALS/ GRAINS** Rice, Millet, Barley, Guinea corn, Acha, Buckwheat, Oat bran, Oat meal, Cassava.	**CEREAS / GRAINS** Maize, Wheat, Semovita, Noodles, Spaghetti, White flower, Cornflakes, Bread (all), Biscuit, Pasta.
VEGETABLES Avocado (Florida) ; Cayenne, Artichoke, Beet green, Greens, Broccoli, Dandelion, Kale, Leek, Okra, Onion, Pumpkin, Parsnip, Lettuce, Romaine, Red pepper, Sweet potato, Kelp, Seaweed, Spinach, Turnip, Parsley.	**VEGETABLES** Beet, Carrot, Celery, Lettuce, Mushroom (Maitake), Green olives, Pepper (green), Radish, Squash, Shallot, Scallion, Yam, Garlic, Chili pepper, Asparagus, Cabbage, Eggplant, Tomato, Green sweet pepper, Red sweet pepper.	**VEGETABLES** Cauliflower, Maize, Cocoyam, Spirulina, Black olive, Mustard green, Irish potato, Alfalfa sprout, Cucumber, Irish potato, Mushroom (Common/ Shiitake/Silver), Avocado (California).

BENEFICIAL FOODS	**NEUTRAL FOODS**	**FOODS TO AVOID COMPLETELY**
FRUITS Fig, Plum, Prune, Banana, Cherry, Blueberry, Guava, Mango.	**FRUITS** Apple, Apricot, Cranberry, Blackcurrant, Date, Starfruit Gooseberry, Grape, Grape fruit, Lemon, Lime, Melon, Pawpaw, Pear, Pineapple, Pomegranate, Tomato, Watermelon, Raisin.	**FRUITS** Blackberry, Cantaloupe, Orange, Plantain, Avocado (California), Kiwi, Bitter Melon, Tangerine.
JUICES Blackberry, Pineapple, Guava, Mango, Prune,	**JUICES** Apricot, Carrot, Celery, Lime, Grapefruit, Pawpaw,	**JUICES** Orange, Aloe, Blackberry, Coconut milk,

Spinach.	Lemon, Cabbage, Tomato, Apple cider, Grape.	Tangerine, Cucumber.
SPICES/CONDIMENTS Carob, Cayenne, Curry, Dulse, Horseradish, Kelp, Parsley, Turmeric, Pepper.	**SPICES/CONDIMENTS** Allspice, Basil, Bergamot, Brown sugar, Chocolate, Coriander, Cumin, Dill, Maple, Marjoram, Molasses, Mustard, Paprika,Peppermint, Rosemary, Sage, Tamarind, Thyme, Vanilla, Cinnamon, Cumin, Clove, Honey, Garlic, Lecithin, Oregano, Brewer's yeast.	**SPICES/CONDIMENTS** MSG, Nutmeg, Pepper (black and white), Aspartame, Corn syrup, Fructose, Ketchup, Vinegar (except apple cider), Sucrose, Mayonnaise, Carragenan, Pickles, Gum Arabic, Cornstarch.
BEVERAGES Green tea, Club soda, Seltzer water.	**BEVERAGES** Red wine	**BEVERAGES** Coffee, Liquor, Beer, Cola Soda, Diet soda, Black tea.
HERBAL TEAS Cayenne, Chickweed, Dandelion, Fenugreek, Ginger, Hops, Linden, Milk thistle, Parsley, Peppermint, Rose hip, Astralagus.	**HERBAL TEAS** Catnip, Chamomile, Ginseng, Valerian, Sage, Thyme, Senna, Peppermint, Skullcap.	**HERBAL TEAS** Aloe vera, Saint-John's wort, Guarana, Corn silk, Echinacea, Black tea (both regular and decaff), Goldenseal, Rhubarb, Shepherd's purse, Strawberry leaf.

APPENDIX B

DR. AFFI'S TEN COMMANDMENTS OF GOOD NUTRITION

1.   Thou shall not poison thyself (avoid fried foods, alcohol, red meat, sugar, processed foods, tinned/canned foods, soft drinks and junk – "junk foods produce junk people")

2.   Thou shall eat 80% of your food raw for life-long vibrant health

3.   Thou shall never miss breakfast – your biggest and richest meal should be your breakfast (Thomas Affi's Breakfast Salad – TABS) highly recommended

4.   Thou shall eat sparingly for a long and disease-free life (eat only ¼ of what you eat at the moment

5.   Thou shall eat according to your blood group

6.   Thou must eat at least five fruits and vegetables daily

7.   Thou shall avoid C.A.T. (Caffeine, Alcohol and Tobacco,)

8.   Thou shall eat little or no red meat as adults and non-pregnant women

9.   Thou shall eat at least four eggs daily (organic; local)

10.   Thou shall eat your supper very early and very light (best eat uncooked food at dinner except for your 2 eggs)

APPENDIX C
DISEASES THAT CAN IMPROVE AND REGRESS WHEN ON THE SUPER-NUTRITION DIET

1.   Addison's Disease
2.   Angina Pectoris
3.   Autoimmune diseases
4.   Stroke
5.   Diabetes Mellitus
6.   Endocrine Diseases
7.   Gallstones
8.   Peptic ulcer disease
9.   Haemorrhoids
10.   Hiatus Hernia
11.   Hypertension
12.   Ischaemic Heart Disease
13.   Irritable Bowel Syndrome
14.   Multiple Sclerosis
15.   Myxoedema
16.   Osteoarthritis
17.   Osteoporosis
18.   Peripheral Vascular Diseases
19.   Pernicious Anaemia
20.   Rheumatoid Arthritis
21.   Senile Dementia
22.   Ulcerative Colitis
23.   Thyrotoxicosis
24.   Varicose Veins

APPENDIX D
THOMAS AFFI'S BREAKFAST SALAD (TABS)

S/N	ITEM	QUANTITY
1	G – Green Leaves	1 cup per person
2	L – Lemon Juice	½ lemon
3	O – Olive Oil	1 tablespoon
4	B – Beet Root	1 cup
5	B – Banana	2 fingers
6	A – Apple Cider Vinegar	1 tablespoon
7	C – Carrot	1 medium
8	C – Cabbage	1 cup
9	A – Avocado	1
10	S – Sunflower Seeds	10g
11	E – Egg	1 hard-boiled
12	B – Beans	1 cup
13	U – – –	
14	S – Sesame (black)	10g
15	T – Tomato	1
16	O – Onions	1 medium
17	P – Pepper (Green/Red)	1
18	S – Starch (Yam/Sweet Potato)	3 medium

MAKE THIS A CHARACTER OF ITS OWN PLEASE

The best lunch ever is a blend of raw fruits, vegetables, nuts, seeds, condiments and spices to build the immunity of the body against infection, cancer and degenerative diseases. The combo provides close to the 91 nutrients that are necessary for conferring longevity and perpetual youthfulness.

These so called "daily-must" drink can literally prevent, control or even cure most common ailments that plague man. For total success, the most crucial aspect of the drink is the acquisition of a good blender or liquidizer. Once you have either of these, your health is guaranteed to remain vibrant for many years to come.

The principle behind the miracle shake is that fact that in nutrition and health, little things go far. It is the little things we throw into our food that always give us the biggest health dividends. When you eat diverse items, you get the entire spectrum of benefits they offer. Simply combining one food with another can make a tremendous difference in your total nutrient intake and offer significant health gain.

1. For instance adding a handful of **Sunflower seeds** or sesame seeds (just ½ cup) to your morning breakfast provides more than 100% of your day's requirement of vitamin E and arginine. Vitamin E and arginine stimulate the pituitary gland to produce hormones that are anti-aging. And vitamin E protects against cancer, heart disease, dementia and Alzheimer's disease.

2. **Red/Green Pepper**: Adding just one medium of red or green pepper provides 100% vitamin C requirement.

3. **Canned Salmon or Sardine or Mackerel:** Eating just3 ounces of any of these provides more than half of your body's weekly requirement of omega -3 fatty acid which is excellent for the heart and brain as well as for the treatment of diabetes mellitus.

4. **Blending Fresh Green Leaves of Spinach** (parboiled) provides 20% daily requirements of vitamin A and lutein that protects against age-related macular disease (ARMD) of the eyes. Eating just 5.8mg of green leaves daily removes the risk of ARMD and cataract.

   Other than blending, another good way of cooking green leaves for health is to stir-fry them meaning you throw in green leaves into red hot "olive oil" and stir for just a few minutes before blending same with other vegetables.

Why you must blend the miracle shake

When vegetables are parboiled, the absorption of nutrients in them improves from 7% to 19%. When they are juiced, absorption further improves from 19% to 100%. Here again lies the vital importance of juicing your vegetables as is done as advocated in TAMS.

APPENDIX F
LEMON BAKED FISH (SPECIAL)

Fish: Use white fish (cod, halibut, dill or turbot) for best results.

Ingredients:

S/N	ITEM	QUANTITY
1	Olive Oil	1 tablespoonful
2	Onion	1 large
3	Lemon	3
4	Fish (White)	2lb (1kg)filled with skin removed
5	Vinegar	1/8 pint of white vinegar
6	Salt	Pinch only
7	Pepper	Fresh ground (black pepper)
8	Butter (fulani)	As relish only
9	Dill	½ teaspoonful
10	Parsley	½ cup

Method:

1. Brush some of the olive oil over the bottom of a shallow baking dish
2. Peel and thinly slice the onion and divide into rings.
3. Very thinly slice the lemon
4. Arrange the sliced onion at the bottom of the baking dish and cover with fish fillets (cut fish into strips of 3 – 4 inches wide if the fish is large)
5. Pour over the vinegar and remaining oil, seasoning with salt and pepper and then top with the slices of lemon.
6. Bake in moderately hot oven at 400^0C/Reg 6 for 20 – 25 minutes until fish is tender.
7. Discard the lemon and onion and reserve the cooking liquid.
8. Arrange the fish on a heated serving dish and warm.
9. Heat the butter over low flame in a saucepan
10. Add chopped dill/parsley and juices from fish and season for a few minutes.

Lemon juice and Green Tea

Addition of the juice of ½ a lemon to a cup of green tea in the morning leads to four fold increase in disease-fighting catechins. Lemon juice is best, but in its absence one can use orange juice, grape fruit or lime juice even though they are less effective.

APPENDIX G

RULES FOR HEALTHFUL EATING

1.   Eat only when you are hungry and even then, use the clock.
2.   Eat no more than the equivalent of two handfuls of food – that's the size of the human stomach.
3.   Do not put any food in your mouth until the previous bite has gone to the stomach-eat very slowly for health
4.   Don't fight natural cravings. If you feel strongly to eat something go ahead and eat it but in very small quantity only to satisfy the urge without damaging your body.
5.   Experience all these six different tastes daily:
a.   Sweet–honey, rice and fish.
b.   Sour–lemons and sour sop.
c.   Salty–sardine, sea salt and pickled olive.
d.   Pungent–ginger, onions, garlic and pepper.
e.   Bitter–spinach, bitter leaf and other green vegetables.
f.   Astringent–beans and turmeric.

Incidentally, all these taste are adequately provided for in the TABS and TAMS, thus, making these two meals truly versatile and all-round for life-long health and vitality.

CHAPTER

THE LIFE EXTENSION PROTOCOL

The maximum lifespan of a man (50 years) may not have changed much over the few millennia but the total number of people approaching it has continued to rise. And the goodness about life extension is that except maybe for one or two high-tech examples, most of the life elongating practices are low-tech and within the reach of most people. For instance some of the most powerful life extension practices like exercise calone restrictions and the consumption of a varied (rainbow) diet of fruits and vegetables are all within the reach of the average man and woman.

For the sake of clarity and brevity, therefore, I have set out below; a checklist of common practices that promote health and longevity and have also added a few of those practices that are inimical to good health. Finally, to encourage active participation, I have provided space on the tables for readers to assess themselves and take appropriate action where necessary; for the name of the game life is "today", as tomorrow may be too late.

The recommended protocol for living vibrantly till ripe old age is as follows:

(1) Physical Exercise protocol:
   a. Do 45 minutes aerobic activity in early morning sunlight (Brisk-walking).
   b. Stretch thoroughly before and after 45 minutes work out.
   c. Use heart rate monitor to make sure you are neither under-nor-over exerting yourself.
   d. Do weight training thrice a week Mondays Wednesdays and Fridays.
   e. Add brisk-walking; dancing, yoga, Tai-chi or Qi-gong.

(2) Nutritional protocol:
   a) Diet and behavioural modification.
   b) Consumption of whole grain foods.
   c) Vitamins, minerals and herbal supplements.
   d) Reduce animal protein to once a week (weekends).
   e) Increase consumption of cold-water fish to 5 times a week (mercury or use cod liver oil)
   f) Increase protein intake from whole grains, legumes, seeds and nuts.
   (3) Fibre: the diet should be provided with at least 45g of fibre per day (T.A.L Diet has double this).

(4) Eat at least 3 servings of cruciferous vegetables daily. Examples of these vegetables are broccoli, cabbage and   cauliflower.

(6) Drink 3 glasses of (blended spinach,   bitter leaf, moringa leaf and ugwu, celery radish, carrots).

(7) Water therapy: As part of the TAL Diet, one is expected to practice regular water drinking to prevent mild chronic dehydration   (MCD)   which is a contributory factor in so many common ailments that humanity. The water therapy protocol is to be done by the odd hours of   the clock as follows:

5:00am: Drink 1,500ml of clean water; gulp down at once while standing or squatting (best).

8:00am: BREAKFAST.

9:00am: top-up with 250ml (sip slowly while sitting)

11:00am: top up of 250ml (sip slowly while sitting)

1:00pm: top up of 250ml (sip slowly while sitting)

3:00pm: top up of 250ml (sip slowly while sitting)

5:00pm: top up of 250ml (sip slowly while sitting)

7:00pm: DINNER

7:00pm: top up of 250ml (sip slowly while sitting) tsp.

9:00pm: BEDTIME cup of chamomile tea+ honey + 1tsp soya bean oil.

This ritual adds up to a total of 3,000ml of water per day which is optimal to guarantee a vibrant, long and healthy life in a hot tropical weather

(8) Avoid junk foods, minerals and soft drinks.

(9) Use extra virgin coconut oil, avocado oil coconut oil and flaxseed oil for all cooking

APPENDIX I
THOMAS AFFI'S DAILY MENU

MEAL	MONDAY	TUESDAY	WEDNESDAY	THURSDAY	FRIDAY	SATURDAY	SUNDAY
BEFORE BREAKFAST	Honey Dates Lemon Juice BSO Acharc Kolanut CIN TMR FEN GIN	Honey Dates Lemon Juice BSO Acharc Kolanut CIN TMR FEN GIN	Honey Dates Lemon Juice BSO Acharc Kolanut CIN TMR FEN GIN	Honey Dates Lemon Juice BSO Acharc Kolanut CIN TMR FEN GIN	Honey Dates Lemon Juice BSO Acharc Kolanut CIN TMR FEN GIN		Honey Dates Lemon Juice BSO Acharc Kolanut CIN TMR FEN GIN
L		Fruits	Fruits	Fruits	Fruits	SABBATH–FASTING	Fruits
	Starch (Root fresh)	Starch (Root fresh)	Starch (Root fresh)	Starch (Root fresh)	Starch (Root fresh)		Starch (Root fresh)
	Proteins Eggs +	Proteins Eggs +	Proteins Eggs +	Proteins Eggs +	Proteins Eggs +		Proteins Eggs +
	Beverages & Condiments Cayenne Ginger Moringa	Beverages & Condiments Cayenne Ginger Moringa	Beverages & Condiments Cayenne Ginger Moringa	Beverages & Condiments Cayenne Ginger Moringa	Beverages & Condiments Cayenne Ginger Moringa		Beverages& Condiments Cayenne Ginger Moringa
	TAMS Swallow	TAMS Swallow	TAMS Swallow	TAMS Swallow	TAMS Swallow		TAMS Swallow

C	millet Guineacorn Oats	millet Guineacorn Oats	millet Guineacorn Oats	millet Guineacorn Oats	millet Guineacorn Oats		millet Guineacorn Oats
	Fruits & Vegetables Fish (Eggs)	Fruits & Vegetables Fish (Eggs)	Fruits & Vegetables Fish (Eggs)	Fruits & Vegetables Fish (Eggs)	Fruits & Vegetables Fish (Eggs)		Fruits & Vegetables Fish (Eggs)
DINNER	Daily-Musts grain starch (brown rice) chamomile Tea Honey 1 tsp soya oil 1 tsp	Daily-Musts grain starch (brown rice) chamomile Tea Honey 1 tsp soya oil 1 tsp	Daily-Musts grain starch (brown rice) chamomile Tea Honey 1 tsp soya oil 1 tsp	Daily-Musts grain starch (brown rice) chamomile Tea Honey 1 tsp soya oil 1 tsp	Daily-Musts grain starch (brown rice) chamomile Tea Honey 1 tsp soya oil 1 tsp		Daily-Musts grain starch (brown rice) chamomile Tea Honey 1 tsp soya oil 1 tsp

BIBLIOGRAPHY

Abdennour, S. (2002). *Egyptian Cooking: A Practical Guide.* The American University In Cairo Press Egypt. 5th Edition.

Abiola, B. (2002). *Indulge In Healthy Living.* Kwagg Publishers South Africa.

Adamo, P.J.D. Dr. and Whitney, C. (1996). *Four Blood Types, Four Diets: Eat Right For Your Type.* Penguin Group New York.

Adodo, A. OSB (2004). *Herbs for Healing.* Benedictine Publication Nigeria. 3rd Edition.

Adodo, A. OSB (2004). *Nature Power.* Benedictine Publication Nigeria. 3rd Edition.

Allen, C., Maleskey, G., Michaud, E., Nuwer, N., Votava L. And Wild, R. (1992). *The Prevention Pain-Relief System.* Rodale Press Emmaus Pennyslyvania.

Allen, C.C. And Winters, C.A. (2004). *The Healthy Balance.* Mindex Publishing Company Limited Edo State, Nigeria.

Anderson, H.L.N. (1990). *Helping Hand: A Guide To Healthy Living for People Who Care About Wellness.* Academy Press Limited Lagos, Nigeria.

Antol, M.N. (1996). Healing Teas: *How to Prepare and Use Teas to Maximize Your Health.* Avery Publishing Groups New York.

Ashton, J. And Ron L. (1998). *The Perils of Progress.* Zeal Books Limited London.

Baikee, P. (1985). *1000 Health and Beauty Hints.* Hennerwood Publications Limited Glasgow.

Bakhru H.K. (2010). *Foods That Heal: The Natural Way to Good Health.* Orients Paperback New Delhi. 2nd Edition.

Bakhru, H.K. (2006). *Vitamins That Heal: Natural Immunity for Better Health.* Orients Paperback New Delhi. 7th Edition.

Balch, P.A. (2003). *Prescription for Dietary Wellness.* Penguin Group Incorporation New York. 2nd Edition.

Benjamin, H.H. And Love, S. (1995). *The Wellness Community: Guide to Fighting for Recovery From Cancer.* Penguin Putnam Incorporation New York.

Berger, S. M.D (1981). *The Southampton Diet.* Pocket Books Press New York.

Bueno, L. (1991). *Fast Your Way To Health.* Whitaker House New Kensington.

Bull, D. (1998). *Vitality Plan.* Dorling Kindersky Limited London.

Cain, A.H (1973). *Young People and Health*John Day Company New York Winick, M (1977) *Nutrition and Cancer.* John Wiley, New York.

Cartland, B. (1976). *The Magic of Honey Cookbook.* Transworld Publishers Limited London.

Castleman, M. (1995). *The Healing Herbs: The Ultimate Guide To The Curative Power   Of Nature's Medicines.* Bantam Books USA. 2nd Edition.

Colbert, D. M.D (2004). *Eat This And Live.* Siloam-A Strang Company, Florida.

Colbert, D. M.D (2004). *What You Don't Know May Be Killing You.* Siloam-A Strang Company,   Florida.

Colbert, D. M.D (2006). *How to Revitalize Your Body In 28 Days.* Mindex Publishing Company   Limited Florida.

Colbert, D. M.D (2006). *Living In Divine Health.* Siloam- A Strang Company Florida.

Cooper, R.K. And Cooper, L.L. (1996). *Low-Fat Living.* Rodale Books USA.

Covey, S.R. (1989). *The Seven Habits to Highly Effective People.* Aviacom Company London.

Cummings, L.E. And Kotschevar, L.H. (1989). *Nutrition Management for Food Services.* DELMAR   Publishers Incorporation, New York.

Dalton, K. (1985). *The Premenstrual Syndrome and Progesterone Therapy.* William Heinemann Medical Books Limited London. 2nd Edition.

Diamond, H. (2003). *Fit For Life Not Fat For Life.* Joint Heirs Publication Limited Nigeria.

Duyff, R.L. (2006). *Complete Food and Nutrition Guide.* John Wiley and Sons Incorporation New Jersey. 3rd Edition.

Eleanox Berman, Heyden, London 1980. *Toxic Metals and their Analysis*

Eric J. Underwood; Academic Press, New York 1977. *Trace Elements in Human and Animal Nutrition*

Eva D. Wilson Ketherine H. Fisher, Mary E. Fugua, John Wiley and Sons. New York, 1959. *Principles of Nutrition*

Feinstein, A., Dollemore, D., Henry, S.J., Holman, M., Kirchheimer, S., Maleskey, G., Pashen, H., Wargo, J. and Wittig, P. (1992). *Training the Body to Cure Itself: How to UseExercise to Heal.* Rodale Press Emmaus Pennsylvania.

Feldman, E.B (1976). *Nutrition and Cardiovascular Disease.* Appleton Century- Crofts, New York.

Feltman, J. (1992). *The Prevention How-To Dictionary Of Healing Remedies And Techniques.* Rodale Press Emmaus Pennyslyvania.

Geddes and Grosset (2005). *Guide to Natural Healing.* Geddes and Grosset Scotland.

Gee, G.E. (1997). *Calculation for Hospitality and Catering.* Holder and Stouhton London. 3rd Edition.

Gotlieb, B. (2008). Alternative Cures.Ballantine Books New York.

Graves, C.P. (1970). *Robert E. Kennedy: Man Who Dared To Dream.* Garrard Publishing Company Illinois.

Gupta, M.K (2009). *Foods That Are Killing You Slowly But Steady.* Pustak Mahal Delhi.

Hauser, G. (1951). *Look Younger, Live Younger.* Faber and Faber Limited London.

Holford, P. And Colson, D. (2008). *Optimum Nutrition for Your Children.* Piakus-Brown Book Group London.

Hubbard, R.L. (1981). *Dianetics:* The Modern Science of Mental Health. Bridge Publications Incorporation California.

Insel, P.M And Roth, W.T. (2006). *Core Concepts in Health.* Mcgraw-Hill Companies Incorporation, New York. 10th Edition.

Joan Gomez George Allen & Unwin Ltd, London 1972.*How Not to Die Young*

John, A.W. (2003). *The Water for Life; a Treatise on Urine Therapy*. The C.W Daniel CompanyLimited England. 13th Edition.

Joshi, S.A. (2002). *Nutrition and Dietetics*. McGraw Hill Publishing Company Limited New Delhi.

Kashiwa, A. and Rippe, J. M.D (1987). *Fitness Walking for Women*. A Perigee Books New York.

Katahn, M. (1989). *The T-Factor Diet*. Bantam Books New York.

Kinderlehrer, J. (1977). *Confessions of a Sneaky Organic Cook*. Rodale Press Incorporation Emmaus Pennyslyvania. 3rd Edition.

Kraut; H.,Oremrr, H.D., Verlag, W (1969). *Investigation intoHealth and Nutrition in East Africa*. Munchen

Kurian, J. (2010). *Healing Wonders of Plants*. Zambia Adventist Press, Zambia. Vol. 1 and 2.

Kurk, M. Dr. and Walker, M. Dr. (1998). *Prescription for Long Life: Essential Remedies for Longevity*. Magna Publishing Company Limited Mumbai.

Labuza, T.P. (1977). *Food and Your Well-Being*. West Publishing Company USA.

Lamb, M.W and Harden, M.L (1973). *The meaning of Nutrition*. Pergamon Press Incorporation.

Lamm, S. M.D (2005). *The Hardness Factor*. Harper Collins Publishers Limited, London.

Laporte, C. (1988). *High Energy Living: How to Put More Zest into Your Life*. WL Books Limited London.

Laurence, E.Mand Gross, L (1975). *Total Fitness*. Hart- DavisMacGibon, London.

Lelord Kodel, W. H. ALLEn, London, 1974. *Natural Folk Remedies*

Levine, G.T. (2007). *Simply Israel: A Collection of Recipes From the People of Isreal*. 2nd Editon.

Lindlahr, H. Dr. (2002). *Nature Cure Healing Without Drugs*. Sterling Publishers Pvt Limited New Delhi.

Lockie, A. Dr. (2001). *Homeopathy Handbook: A Potent Force to Help Overcome Illness and Fight Disease.* A Dorling Kindersley Book.

Lunden, J and Winick, J. M.D (2004). *Growing Up Healthy: a Complete Guide to Childhood Nutrition, Birth Through Adolescence.* Atria Books New York.

Mallos, T. (1993). *The Complete Middle East Cookbook.* Lansdowne Publishing Pty Limited Australia.

Manger, W., Kaplan, N., Roccella, E.J. And Late Dr. Gifford, R.W. Jnr (2011). *101 Questions and Answers about Hypertension.* Kiran S. Rana. 2nd Edition.

Medical Glossary (1998). *Vitamins and Mineral: Health, Diet, Fighting Disease.* Medical. Geddes and Grosset Limited Scotland.

Melgosa, J. (2012). *Enjoy Life: A Practical Guide To Living Better And Longer.* Safeliz S.L. Spain. 1st Edition.

Merki, M.B. And Merki, D. (1987). *A Guide to Wellness.* Glencoe Publishing Company California.

Michaud, E. And Wild, R. (2010). *How to Boost Your Brain Power.* Self Improvement Publishing, Benin City, Nigeria.

Miller, C. (1986). Fred'n'Erma. Intervarsity Press Illinois.

Minirth, F., Krusz, J.C., Hopewell, A. And Neal, V. (2005). *The Christian Guide to Natural Products and Remedies.* Broadman and Holman Publishers, Tennessee.

Mitchell, C., Baildam, E., Bull, D., Clemonds A., And Marshall, D. (2003). *Vibrant Health In The 21st Century.* The Stanborough Press Limited England. 5th Edition.

Molnar, E. Michael M.D. (2005) *Forever Young II. The Fundamentals of a 'Younger Longer' Life.* Stem Cell Transplantation Project for Africa.

Momoh-Aliu, B. ND (2007). *Foods and Herbs for Radiant Health And Spiritual Ascent.* CSS Bookshop Limited Lagos Nigeria.

Noder, W. M.D (1983). *Speaking of Fitness Over 40.* Sterling Publishers Pvt Limited New Delhi.

Obeki, O.S. (2007). *Fat Or Thin: Facts And Counsel On Weight Loss And Weight Gain.* Mindex Press Benin City Nigeria.

Ojo, O. (2007). *The Secrets of Longevity.* New Round Agencies Limited Abuja Nigeria.

Ojo, O. (2009). *Natural Beauty Secrets.* New Round Agencies Limited Abuja Nigeria.

Ojofeitimi, E.O. (2007). *Principles and Practices of Nutrition For Community Health Workers.* Nonesuchhouse Publishers. 3rd Edtion.

Okokoh, L. Dr. (2005). *Foods That Heal; Foods That Kill.* Capstone Natural Health CentreLimited Lagos, Nigeria. 1st Edition.

Padus, E. (1992). *The Complete Guide to Your Emotions And Your Health.* Rodale Press Emmaus Pennyslyvania.

Pamplona-Roger,G.D. M.D (2001). *Encyclopedia of Foods and Their Healng Power.* MARPAArtes Graficas Spain. Vol 1,2 and 3.

Pamplona-Roger, G.D. M.D (2004). *Encyclopedia of Medicinal Plants.* Safeliz S.L. Spain. Vol. 1and 2; 7th Edition.

Pamplona-Roger, G.D. M.D (2010). *Healthy Body: A Practical Guide to Body Care.* Safeliz S.L. Spain. 2nd Edition.

Pamplona-Roger, G.D. M.D (2010). *Healthy Foods.* Graficas Estella Spain. 1st Edition.

Pamplona-Roger, G.D. M.D And Malaxetxebarria, E. M.D (2007). *250 Recipes for Healing and Prevention.* Safeliz S.L. Spain. 1st Edition.

Pasternak, H. And Murphy, M. (2006). *The Five (5) Factor Diet.* Meredith Books Iowa.

Poskitt, E.M.E. (1988). *Practical Peadiatric Nutrition.* Butterworth Company Ands Publishers Limited.

Pritikin, N. And Mcgrady, P.M. Jr. (1981). *The Pritikin Program for Diet And Exercise.* Bantam Books Incorporation New York.

Randolph, C.W.M.D and James, G. (2008). *From Belly Fat to Belly Flat.* Health Communications Incorporation, Deerfield Beach.

Richard J.B.W. (2001). *Your Health In Your Hands.* The Stanborough Press Limited England. 6th Edition.

Robert H. Williams, Springer-Verlagi New York, 1973. *To Live and To Die*

Rogers, J. (2001). *The Bibles Seven Secrets to Healthy Eating.* Crossway Books, Illinois.

Roizen, M.F And Mehmet, C. Oz, M.D (2006). *You on a Diet.* Free Press New York.

Schneider, E. Dr. (2004). *Healthy By Nature.* Artes Graficas Toledo Spain. 1st Edition.

Sofowora, A. (2012). *Medicinal Plants and Traditional Medicine in Africa.* Spectrum Books LimitedIbadan Nigeria.

Swartout, H.O. M.D (1945). *Modern Medical Counselor: A Practical Guide to Health.* Pacific Press Publishing Association California.

Tenney, D. (1992). *An Introduction to Natural Health.* Woodland Books USA.

Tension, M.H. (1974). *Eat Well and Be Slim.* Pan Books Limited London.

The Editors of FC and A (2008). *Healthy, Wealthy And Wise.* FC and A Publishing USA.

The Editors of FC and A (2008). *Super Foods for Senior.* FC and A Publishing USA.

The Staff of Prevention Magazine (1976). *The Encyclopedia Of Common Diseases.* Rodale Press Incorporation USA.

Tsarice, J.E, M.D And Jonah, K. (1986). *The Palm Beach Long-Life Diet.* Pocket Books Press New York.

Verhulst, D. M.D (2012). *Do This and Live Healthy.* Siloam-A Strang Company Florida.

Vermon S.B., Hirst, C.C. And Jensen, R.K. (1972). *Conditioning Exercises: Exercise to Improve Body Form and Function.* The C.V Mosby Company USA. 3rd Editon.

Vodka, P. (2006). *Exercising for a Healthy Heart.* Orient Paperbacks New Delhi. 6th Edition.

Walia, M.M. (2006). *Stress-Free Living: A Unique Guide To Stress-Free Living.* New Dawn Press Group India. 2nd Edition.

Walker, M. Dr. (1994). *Sexual Nutrition.* Instant Improvement Incorporation New York.

Warren, R., Amen, D., Hyman, M., Foy, S. And Eastman, D. (2013). *The Daniel Plan-40 Days to Healthier Life.* Zondervan, USA.

Weil, A. M.D (2005). *Healthy Aging: A Lifelong Guide to Your Well-Being.* Anchor Books New York.

White, E.G. (1951). *Counsels on Health and Instruction to Medical Missionary Workers.* Pacific Press Publishing Association California. 2nd Edition.

Wright, K. (2002). *Extend Your Life, Nutrition And Supplements: Conventional And Complementary Medicine.* Geddes and Grosset Scotland.

Wright, K. (2005). *Healing Foods: Description, Properties, Health Benefits.* Geddes and Grosset Scotland.

Zelicoff, A. M.D and Michael, B. (2008). *More Harm than Good.* AMACOM New York.

Zinczenko, D. And Spiker, T. (2004). *The Abs Diet: the 6-Week Plan to Flatten Your Stomachand Keep You Lean for Life.* Rodale International Limited   London.